Y0-BDP-109

3 9502 00128 6970

YA   The eyes and
617.7   mouth
Rea

Clark Public Library
303 Westfield Ave.
Clark, NJ 07066
(732)388-5999

EYES
THE
&MOUTH

YOUR BODY YOUR HEALTH

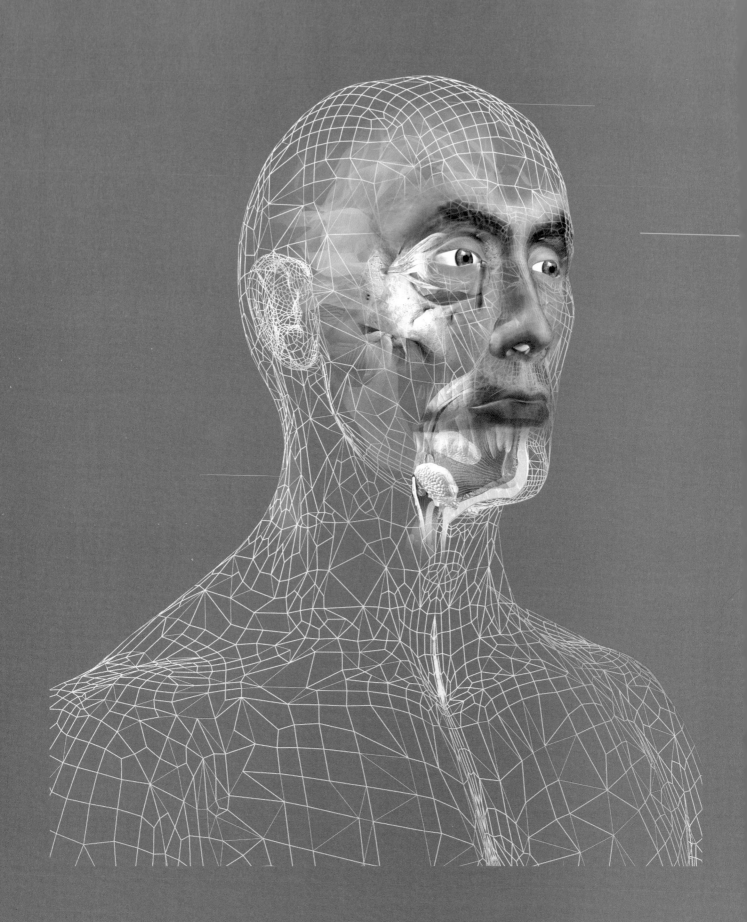

THE EYES & MOUTH

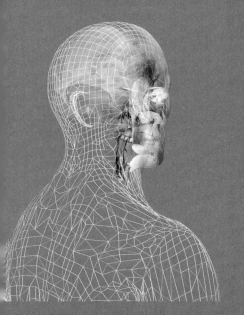
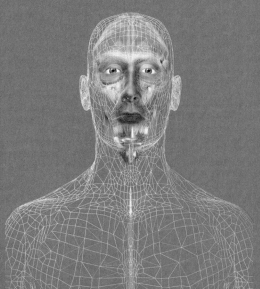
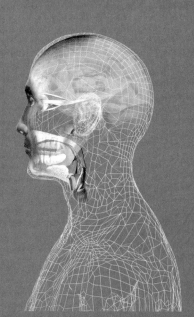

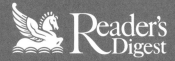

Reader's Digest

The Reader's Digest Association, Inc.

Pleasantville, New York

London Sydney Montreal

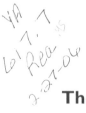

YA
617. 7
617 Rea
3-27-04

The Eyes and Mouth

was created and produced by
Carroll & Brown Limited
20 Lonsdale Road
London NW6 6RD
for Reader's Digest, London

First English Edition Copyright © 2003
The Reader's Digest Association Limited
London

Copyright © 2003 The Reader's Digest
Association, Inc.

All rights reserved.
No part of this book may be reproduced, stored
in a retrieval system or transmitted in any form
or by any means, electronic, electrostatic,
magnetic tape, mechanical, photocopying,
recording or otherwise, without permission in
writing from the publishers.

® Reader's Digest, The Digest and the
Pegasus logo are registered trademarks of
The Reader's Digest Association Inc. of
Pleasantville, New York, USA.

Library of Congress Cataloging-in-Publication Data
The eyes and mouth / Reader's Digest.–
1st American ed.
p. cm. – (Your body, your health)
Includes index.
ISBN 0-7621-0531-3 (Hardcover)
1. Eye–Popular works. 2. Eye–Care and hygiene–
Popular works. 3. Eye–Diseases–Treatment–
Popular works. 4. Mouth. 5. Mouth–Care and
hygiene–Popular works. 6. Mouth–Diseases–
Treatment–Popular works.
I. Reader's Digest Association. II. Series.
RE51.E946 2003
617.7–dc22
2003021386

Printed in the United States of America
1 3 5 7 9 8 6 4 2

The information in this book is for reference only; it is not intended as a substitute for a doctor's diagnosis and care. The editors urge anyone with continuing medical problems or symptoms to consult a doctor.

American Edition Produced by
NOVA Graphic Services, Inc.
2370 York Road, Suite A9A
Jamison, PA 18929 USA
(215) 542-3900

President
David Davenport

Editorial Director
Robin C Bonner

Composition Manager
Steve Magnin

Associate Project Editor
Linnea Hermanson

Otolaryngology Specialist Consultant
Dr Milan Amin, MD
Drexel University College of Medicine/Hahneman Medical College, Philadelphia

CONTRIBUTORS

Wynnie Chan, BSc, PhD, Public Health Nutritionist

Dr Sandeep H Cliff, MB, BSc, MRCP, Consultant Dermatologist,
Honorary Senior Lecturer, Surrey

Mr Brian Coghlan, MD, FRCS (Plast), Consultant Plastic Surgeon, Guy's Hospital, London

F J Cunningham, MRIPH MIT (Lond), Member of the Institute of Trichologists,
The Trichology Centre, Rochdale

Christel Edwards-de Graauw, Nail Technician, Nail Artist and Makeup Artist,
Fingernails Direct, Northern Ireland

Dr Colin Fleming, BSc, MB ChB, MRCP,
Consultant Dermatologist, Department of Dermatology, Ninewells Hospital, Dundee,
Honorary Senior Lecturer, University of Dundee

Katy Glynne, BSc, MRPharmS, Dip Pharmacy Practice,
Clinical Services Manager, Charing Cross Hospital, London,
Clinical Lecturer, The School of Pharmacy, University of London

Dr Lesley Hickin, MB BS, BSc, DRCOG, MRCGP, General Practitioner

Dr Shona Ogilvie, MB ChB, MRCGP, Clinical Fellow,
University Department of Dermatology, Ninewells Hospital, Dundee

Penny Preston, MB ChB, MRGCP, Medical Writer

Beverly Westwood, RN, BSc, MSc, Research Director to Mr Brian Coghlan

For Reader's Digest
Editor in Chief and Publishing Director Neil E Wertheimer
Managing Editor Suzanne G Beason
Production Technology Manager Douglas A Croll
Manufacturing Manager John L Cassidy
Production Coordinator Leslie Ann Caraballo

Clark Public Library - Clark, N. J.

The Eyes and Mouth

Awareness of health issues and expectations of medicine are greater today than ever before. A long and healthy life has come to be looked on as not so much a matter of luck but as almost a right. However, as our knowledge of health and the causes of disease has grown, it has become increasingly clear that health is something that we can all influence, for better or worse, through choices we make in our lives. *Your Body Your Health* is designed to help you make the right choices to make the most of your health potential. Each volume in the series focuses on a different physiological system of the body, explaining what it does and how it works. There is a wealth of advice and health tips on diet, exercise and lifestyle factors, as well as the health checks you can expect throughout life. You will find out what can go wrong and what can be done about it, and learn from people's real-life experiences of diagnosis and treatment. Finally, there is a detailed A to Z index of the major conditions which can affect the system. The series builds into a complete user's manual for the care and maintenance of the entire body.

This volume looks at two of the body's most amazing organs, the eyes and mouth. Discover how your eyes take in visual information from the world around you and the vital role that your brain plays in your ability to see. Find out how taste works, how your mouth forms sounds and how the structure of your teeth makes them uniquely suited to their essential role in eating and digestion. A clear understanding of how the eyes work and how they change with age can help you to spot problems early and get appropriate treatment. Teeth will last a lifetime if they are cared for effectively so regular cleaning techniques are described. A healthy diet builds strong teeth and fights decay while preserving night vision, so read what to eat for optimal health in these organs. Even if eyes and teeth do suffer trauma, there's a lot that can be done to preserve useful vision and to strengthen or replace missing teeth: discover your choices and the pros and cons of each, and meet the whole team of professionals who work to prevent, diagnose and treat problems.

Contents

How your eyes and mouth work

2 Keeping your eyes and mouth healthy

TAKE CHARGE OF YOUR HEALTH

GOOD HEALTH FOR THE EYES AND MOUTH

DIET AND THE EYES AND MOUTH

3

What happens when things go wrong

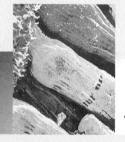

The life story of the eyes and mouth

The eyes and mouth are two of the body's major sensory organs. The eyes enable you to take in information about the world around you, helping you appreciate the world's greatest literature and its most awe-inspiring scenery. Your mouth savors a fine wine and a shrimp scampi meal and allows you to form sounds—a fundamental of human communication.

People have always been fascinated by the eyes, often described as the "windows to the soul."

In the fifth century B.C., the philosopher Empedocles claimed that sight emanated from a fire lit by the Greek goddess of love, Aphrodite, burning within the eyes,. For many years, people continued to believe that this vital sense originated within the eyes themselves. It wasn't until A.D. 1000 that the Arab scientist Ibn al-Haytham put forward a theory that sight was the result of objects reflecting light rays from the sun into the eyes.

About 600 years later, German scientist Johann Kepler provided the first correct explanation of how the human eye works, including how an upside-down image is formed on the retina. Since then, we have come to understand the workings of the eye more clearly and how the information it receives is processed in the brain.

The eye is a highly symbolic organ and is found in many symbols and charms around the world. Throughout the Mediterranean region, for example, an eye symbol can be seen on jewelry, above doorways, and on ships. This ancient symbol is still believed by many to protect against the evil eye—the belief that someone can bring illness or other misfortune to another person through a jealous or spite-filled stare.

FOOD FOR THOUGHT

Like the eye, the mouth is essential to most of the moves we make. First and foremost, it takes in the food we need to fuel our activities and begins the process of digesting it. The mouth plays a crucial role in communication, transforming sounds generated in the throat into recognizable speech. Through specialized nerve endings located on the tongue and in the lining of the mouth, it provides us with the sensations—and pleasures—of taste.

The art of communication
We communicate by more than words. Our body language, including the way we look at each other, conveys a great deal about how we feel and think. In many cultures, the belief persists that a hostile look can bring misfortune, and the ancient eye symbol—seen here on a traditional fishing boat (inset)—is worn for protection and luck.

SEEING THE LIGHT

Light rays enter the front of the eye and pass through structures that bend them the right amount so that they meet on the retina, the light-sensitive area at the back of the eye. This bending of light is called refraction, and most of it occurs as the light passes through the lens at the front of the eye. The lens itself can change its shape—and therefore its power—as appropriate, to ensure that light rays focus on the retina.

MAKING SENSE

The images formed on the retina are actually upside-down. It is the brain that makes sense of images so that we see things the right way up. The retina converts the light rays into electrical impulses, which are sent via the optic nerve to the visual cortex of the brain for processing. Because there are millions of connections between the visual cortex and other parts of the brain, vision is able to play a crucial role in our decisions and actions.

The brain also plays a key role in the sensation of taste, which contributes so much to our enjoyment of food and drink. Specialized nerve endings in the mouth called taste buds are bombarded with different flavors whenever we have anything to eat or drink. As with vision and the other senses, this information is transmitted along nerves as electrical impulses to the brain for processing. Our perception of tastes is strongly influenced by another of our senses: smell.

BEGINNING THE JOURNEY

Before food can be used for fuel by the cells of the body, it must undergo digestion, a series of processes that break down food into its simplest constituent parts. Digestion begins in the mouth with mechanical breakdown (the teeth chew, cut, and grind the food into smaller pieces) and chemical breakdown (a chemical in saliva begins the breakdown of carbohydrates). The tongue, which is also the main site of taste buds, moves the food around the mouth and shapes each mouthful into a ball of food, known as a bolus, suitable for swallowing.

The optic nerve is rather like a cable of electrical wires, made up of about 1.2 million separate tiny wires, or nerve fibers.

THE DEVELOPING EYE

The eyes begin to develop very early in pregnancy; by the end of the fourth week, they have begun to emerge as tiny pouches on each side of the developing brain. The outer part expands, while the part near the brain narrows; at this early stage of its development, the eye is the shape of a lollipop. As it continues to develop, the bulbous end becomes indented and the structure takes on a goblet shape. This "goblet" will form the nerve tissue of the eye. Gradually, other embryonic tissue develops into the lens and the various other parts of the eye.

The eyelids form after about 6 weeks as tiny skin folds. They come together to cover the cornea after 10 weeks and remain closed until the fetus is about 6 months old.

FROM DAY 1

Newborn babies have poor vision; they can probably make out shapes but not much color. This is for two reasons: Although the retina is in place, it is not yet developed, and the visual part of the brain (the visual cortex) is immature. The retina completes its development by the age of 6 weeks or more; the visual cortex takes longer. The nerve

Eyes wide shut
By the eighth week of development, a fetus's eyes have a lens and retina; 2 weeks later teeth start to form in the gums. By 30 weeks—the age of the fetus on this ultasound image—the eyes are fully formed, with lashes and parted lids.

A LIFETIME FOR THE EYES AND MOUTH

The eyes undergo vast changes as we age, sharpening from birth into childhood but changing in middle age. The teeth are completely replaced once, and, with good oral health they can last a lifetime.

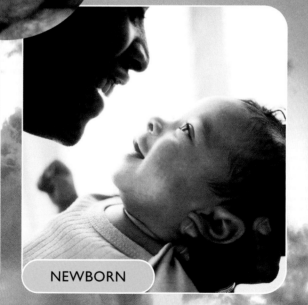

NEWBORN

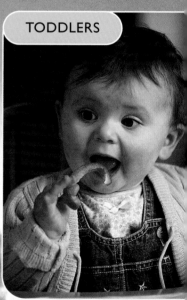

TODDLERS

Holding power
A newborn baby can probably only make out shapes. During the weeks after birth, the ability to recognize faces and features gradually develops.

Taste it and see
By 1 year old, most children have at least one or two teeth that enable them to experiment with more tastes and textures.

A young adult has about 10,000 taste buds, but by the mid-40s, this number has started to decline: It is thought that this reduction does not necessarily affect our ability to differentiate flavors.

tissue in this part of the brain develops rapidly for the first 2 years of life and continues to develop more slowly until about 8 years old. During this time, nerve connections are forming and being reinforced by the constant flow of information from the outside world. Gradually, the baby learns to use visual information, along with information from the other senses, to form an impression of the world.

AS TIME GOES BY
Throughout life, the lens continues to grow. However, by the time we are about 45 years old, it has lost much of its

elasticity, making it difficult for us to focus on close objects. This is why so many middle-aged and older people need to wear reading glasses. This condition is called presbyopia, and it is a natural part of the aging process. Distance vision is unaffected by this change.

By the age of about 60 years, the lens is yellowish in color rather than completely clear, as it is when we are younger. This affects the light rays that can pass through the lens to focus on the retina, causing our color perception of the world to change. This, too, is a normal part of the aging process.

Mix and match
The jaw grows from birth, so that by the age of 6, when the first teeth start to fall out, it can accommodate the larger permanent teeth. Most children have lost all of their first teeth by the age of 12.

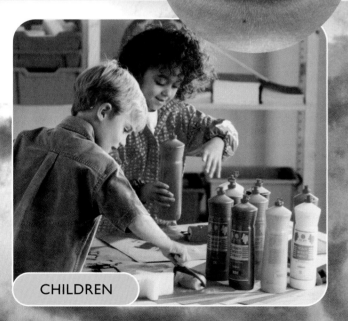

CHILDREN

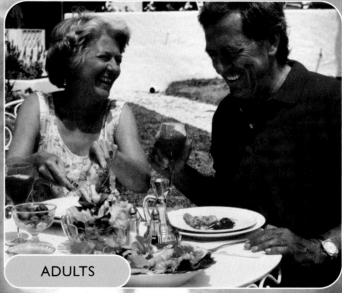

ADULTS

Riot of color
The eyes feed young children's voracious appetite for information about the world around them. By the age of about 3, most children can recognize and name colors.

A feast for the senses
Good food is a feast for the eyes as well as the taste buds. The sight—and smell—of appetizing food trigger the salivary glands to produce saliva, prompting the digestive process.

THE DEVELOPING MOUTH

The first signs of the developing face are five prominences, or swellings, in the upper part of the embryo. The paired maxillary and mandibular prominences lie above and below what becomes the mouth opening. Initially, this opening is sealed off from the amniotic cavity by a membrane, but by the end of week 4, the membrane splits open and the embryo can then swallow amniotic fluid. The prominences undergo a series of fusion processes that bring them together to form the various parts of the face and mouth, including the maxilla (part of the upper jaw), the mandible (lower jaw), and the palate. The palate then develops into the hard palate (at the front of the mouth) and the soft palate (at the back). Failure of the prominences to fuse correctly during fetal development results in facial abnormalities, such as a cleft palate and cleft lip. Today, surgical repair of such defects is usually very successful.

THE FIRST INSTINCT

The instinct to suckle comes naturally to a baby, enabling it to take in milk, its sole food for several months. Simply stroking a newborn baby's cheek stimulates the baby to turn toward you with mouth open, ready to suckle. This primitive response is known as the rooting reflex, and it usually disappears in the first few months.

PROTECTING YOUR MOUTH

Tooth decay is a common problem, affecting most people at some time in their lives. However, it is not inevitable: Avoiding sugary foods and following a program of regular brushing and flossing reduce the risk of cavities.

It is worth remembering that tooth decay is not the only problem that can affect teeth. Many people suffer from gum inflammation (gingivitis), which in its most severe form may result in erosion of the underlying bone and eventual tooth loss. The risks of gum disease are reduced by careful brushing and flossing to remove debris and plaque from between the teeth and along the gum line. Regular visits to a dentist are recommended to help keep the teeth and gums as clean as possible.

Lifestyle is another important factor in looking after the health of your mouth. Smoking, chewing tobacco, and drinking excessive amounts of alcohol are all risk factors for mouth disorders, including oral cancer. In certain parts of India, oral cancer is common because of the practice of chewing tobacco and betel nuts, another risk factor.

Light sensitive at all ages
In this false-colored scanning electron micrograph, light-sensitive rods in the retina are colored orange and the color-sensitive cones are blue. Cone numbers decline as we age, but this appears to have little effect on visual acuity.

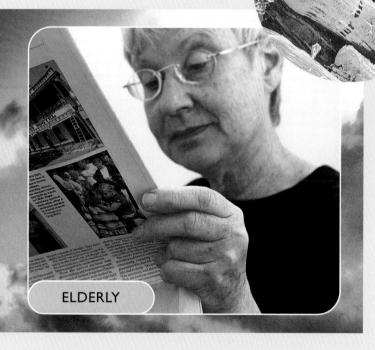

ELDERLY

Spectacle support
For most of us, the eyes play a key role in maintaining quality and enjoyment of life. Some gradual deterioration of vision is to be expected, but this can usually be corrected adequately by glasses or contact lenses.

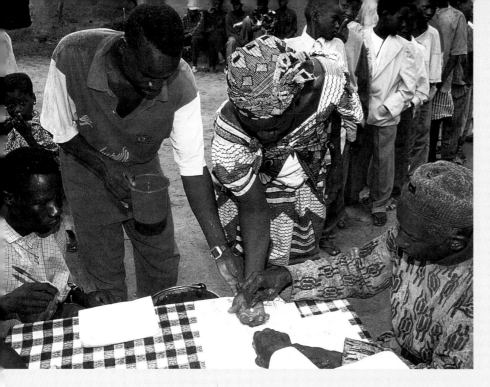

Saving sight

Many of the major causes of blindness in the third world are treatable, often with simple antibiotics. Here, a group of patients in Mali receives antibiotics against river blindness, the world's second leading cause of infection-related sight loss.

BLINDNESS: A MAJOR THIRD-WORLD PROBLEM

It has been estimated that about 50 million people in the world are blind and that in more than half of these cases, the blindness could be reversed. One of the main causes of reversible blindness around the world is cataracts, cloudy areas in the normally transparent lens of the eye. As these opacities thicken, they reduce the amount of light rays passing through the lens to the retina. If the condition is left untreated, blindness is often the eventual result.

In most cases, cataracts can be treated with surgery. In the developing world, however, cataracts remain a major problem because of lack of access to this surgery. A number of organizations are sending teams of surgeons into third-world countries with the aim of treating as many people as they can.

Night blindness resulting from long-term vitamin A deficiency is also common, as is trachoma, a persistent eye infection caused by the chlamydia organism. Although trachoma is rare in developed countries, it is a serious cause of blindness in parts of the world where there is poor sanitation and limited access to the antibiotics needed to treat it. It is estimated that about 6 million people worldwide are blind as a result of trachoma.

LOOKING AHEAD—LASER TREATMENT

Lasers are a more recent tool found to have a role in vision correction. They can be used to treat both near- and farsightedness by reshaping the cornea to be either flatter or more curved. This affects how the light rays entering the eye are bent, enabling them to meet as they should on the retina. In many cases, corrective lenses are no longer needed after laser treatment.

A WINNING SMILE

Many treatments are now available to improve not just the function but also the appearance of teeth. Cosmetic dentistry to whiten teeth by bleaching, to replace missing teeth by implants, and to repair chipped teeth are increasingly common. Teeth can also be repositioned and straightened through the dental specialty of orthodontics, which uses corrective appliances, sometimes over a period of years.

Retinal implants: the way ahead?

An implant mimics the human retina: Light is converted into electrical impulses, which travel along the optic nerve to the brain. In this image, the light-sensitive areas of the implant (center), attached to a human neuron (the dark spot), pick up light (paler areas).

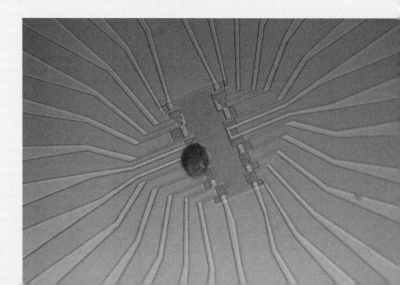

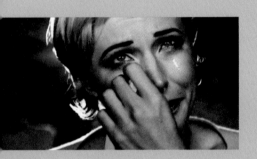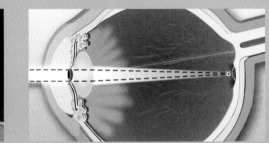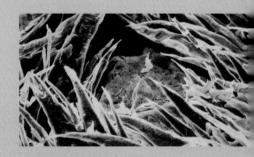

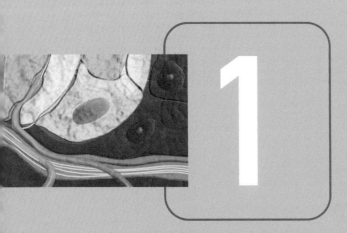

1

How your eyes and mouth work

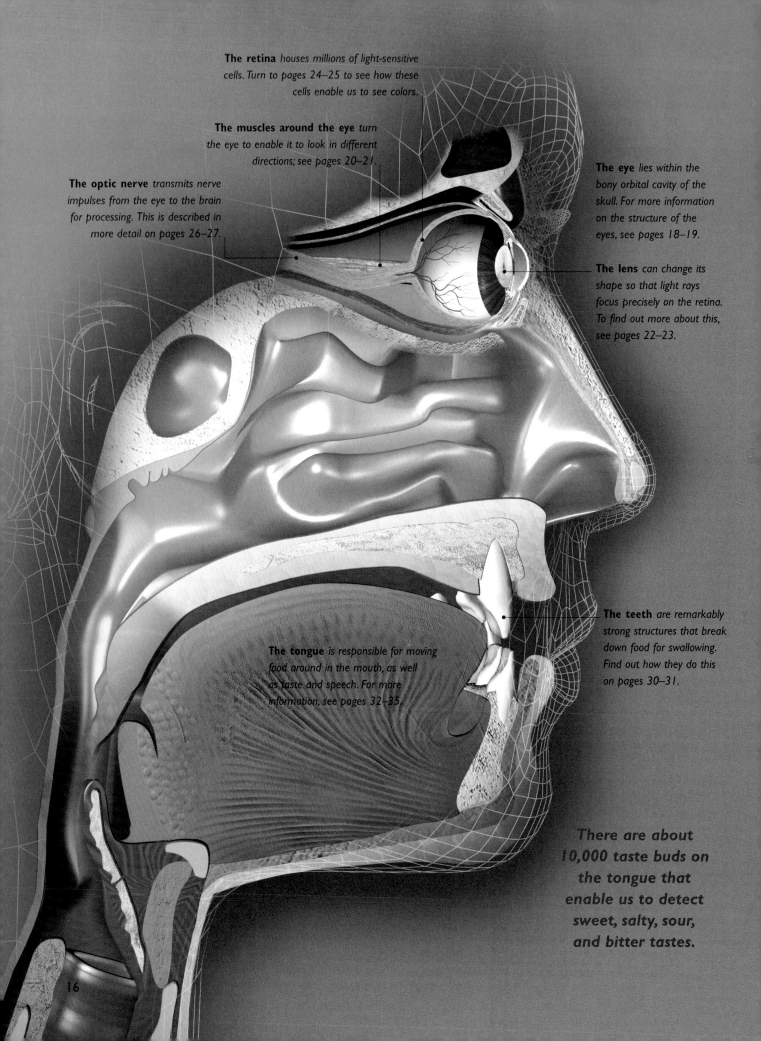

The retina houses millions of light-sensitive cells. Turn to pages 24–25 to see how these cells enable us to see colors.

The muscles around the eye turn the eye to enable it to look in different directions; see pages 20–21.

The optic nerve transmits nerve impulses from the eye to the brain for processing. This is described in more detail on pages 26–27.

The eye lies within the bony orbital cavity of the skull. For more information on the structure of the eyes, see pages 18–19.

The lens can change its shape so that light rays focus precisely on the retina. To find out more about this, see pages 22–23.

The teeth are remarkably strong structures that break down food for swallowing. Find out how they do this on pages 30–31.

The tongue is responsible for moving food around in the mouth, as well as taste and speech. For more information, see pages 32–33.

There are about 10,000 taste buds on the tongue that enable us to detect sweet, salty, sour, and bitter tastes.

Your amazing eyes and mouth

For most of us, the eyes provide our most important information source on the world about us, enabling us to see objects and colors and to judge distances. The mouth provides us with our sense of taste, helps us communicate, and takes in the food that fuels our activities.

YOUR WINDOW ON THE WORLD

Yours eyes are remarkable. Throughout your waking hours, light rays reflected by objects around you are focused on the retina, at the back of your eye. This triggers electrical impulses, which travel along nerves to the brain to be processed, enabling you to see. In the following pages, we will look at the structure of these delicate organs, how they are protected within their sockets, and how they move, providing a panoramic view.

Thanks to the eyes' ability to adjust, we are able to see not only near and far objects, but also in bright and dim light. We can see in glorious technicolor, because of the different light-sensitive cells in the retina. Finally, we will look at how the information received by the eyes in the form of light rays is processed to give us our view of the world.

A GRAND ENTRANCE

The mouth is food's first port of call on its journey through the digestive tract. It is here that food is broken down into smaller pieces ready te be swallowed and where the complex process of digestion begins. The palate (the roof of the mouth) and the movements of the lips and tongue also play a vital role in speech, and thousands of taste buds on the tongue and in the lining of the mouth enable us to detect and enjoy many different tastes and flavors.

We will look at the structure of the mouth and what lies within it and show how it performs its various functions. In particular, we will examine the teeth and how they are specifically designed to fulfill different roles.

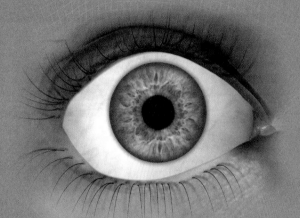

The iris *gives the eye its color, as is described on pages 18–19.*

The pupil, *at the center of the eye, adjusts its size according to the level of brightness and the distance from an object. For more information on how this is done, see pages 22–23.*

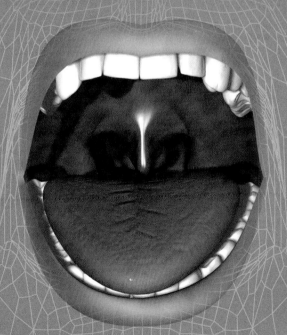

The various parts of the mouth *work together and separately to fulfill the mouth's vital functions of eating and communicating. To find out more about these structures and how they operate, see pages 28–35.*

Inside the eye

The eye converts light rays reflected from objects in front of us into messages that can be processed and interpreted by the brain. The various structures of the eye work together to achieve this.

MAKING LIGHT WORK

When you look at an object, the light rays reflected by that object pass through the front part of your eye and are bent to meet precisely on the back wall of your eye—the retina. The nerve impulses that this produces are passed to the brain, where they are processed into the images that you see before you.

The optic nerve *contains the nerve fibers that transmit impulses to the brain for processing. Blood vessels that accompany the optic nerve branch when they reach the eye to deliver blood to and drain it from the retina.*

The macula lutea *is a circular spot—about 1/5-inch across—that marks the location of the greatest number of light-sensitive cones on the retina.*
The fovea centralis, *at the center of the macula lutea, is where light rays focused on the retina produce the clearest, sharpest image.*

The sclera *is a continuation of the cornea. Seen from the front as the white of the eye, this layer protects the contents of the eye.*

The choroid *lies beneath the sclera. It contains blood vessels that supply and drain blood from the eye.*

The retina *is the innermost layer of the eye and is extremely delicate. It is here that light rays meet (are focused) after entering the eye. Light-sensitive cells in the retina, called rods and cones, convert light rays into nerve impulses that are transported to the brain for processing.*

Vitreous humor *fills the part of the eye behind the lens. It is a jellylike substance composed mainly of water.*

EYE COLOR

The color of the eyes is determined by the amount of pigment in the iris. If the pigment is very concentrated, the eyes appear brown. If only a small amount of pigment is present, the eyes appear blue, green, or gray. All babies are born with blue eyes; their final eye color takes a few months to emerge.

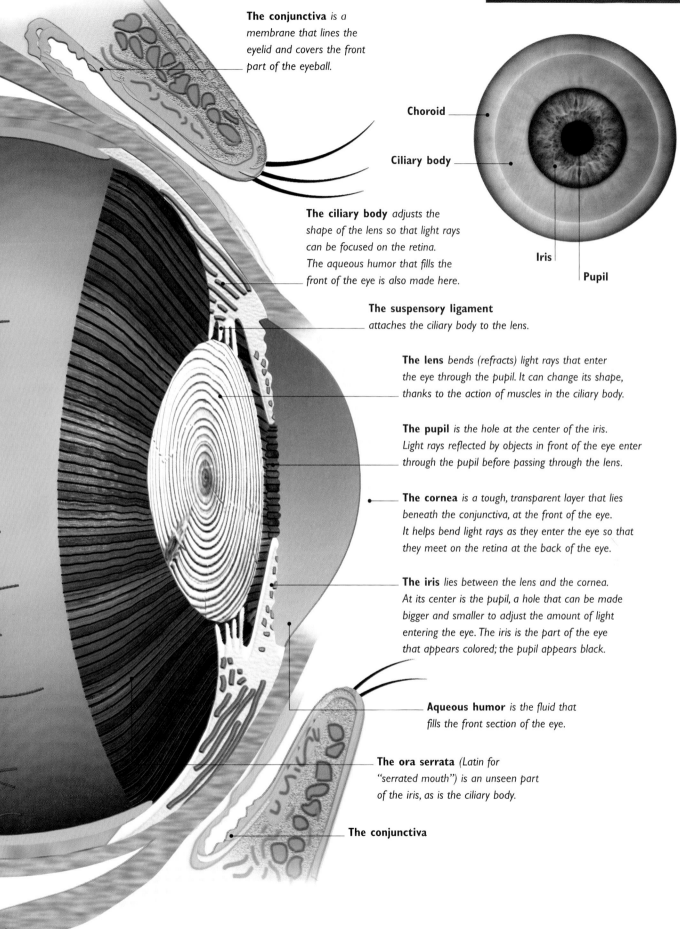

The conjunctiva *is a membrane that lines the eyelid and covers the front part of the eyeball.*

Choroid

Ciliary body

Iris

Pupil

The ciliary body *adjusts the shape of the lens so that light rays can be focused on the retina. The aqueous humor that fills the front of the eye is also made here.*

The suspensory ligament *attaches the ciliary body to the lens.*

The lens *bends (refracts) light rays that enter the eye through the pupil. It can change its shape, thanks to the action of muscles in the ciliary body.*

The pupil *is the hole at the center of the iris. Light rays reflected by objects in front of the eye enter through the pupil before passing through the lens.*

The cornea *is a tough, transparent layer that lies beneath the conjunctiva, at the front of the eye. It helps bend light rays as they enter the eye so that they meet on the retina at the back of the eye.*

The iris *lies between the lens and the cornea. At its center is the pupil, a hole that can be made bigger and smaller to adjust the amount of light entering the eye. The iris is the part of the eye that appears colored; the pupil appears black.*

Aqueous humor *is the fluid that fills the front section of the eye.*

The ora serrata *(Latin for "serrated mouth") is an unseen part of the iris, as is the ciliary body.*

The conjunctiva

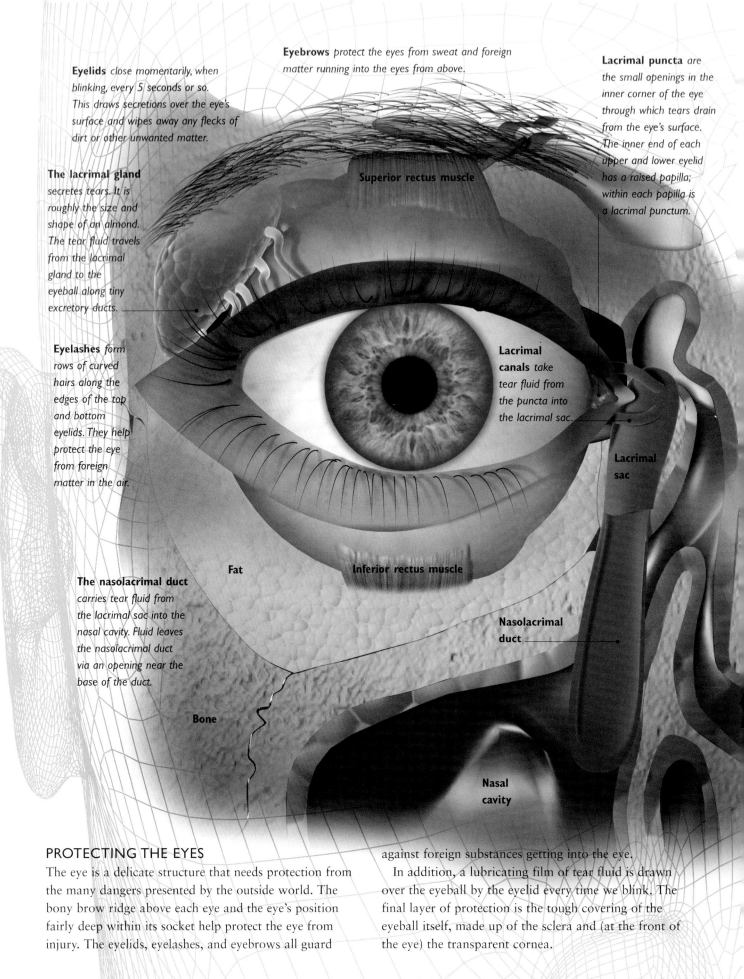

Eyelids close momentarily, when blinking, every 5 seconds or so. This draws secretions over the eye's surface and wipes away any flecks of dirt or other unwanted matter.

Eyebrows protect the eyes from sweat and foreign matter running into the eyes from above.

Lacrimal puncta are the small openings in the inner corner of the eye through which tears drain from the eye's surface. The inner end of each upper and lower eyelid has a raised papilla; within each papilla is a lacrimal punctum.

The lacrimal gland secretes tears. It is roughly the size and shape of an almond. The tear fluid travels from the lacrimal gland to the eyeball along tiny excretory ducts.

Superior rectus muscle

Eyelashes form rows of curved hairs along the edges of the top and bottom eyelids. They help protect the eye from foreign matter in the air.

Lacrimal canals take tear fluid from the puncta into the lacrimal sac.

Lacrimal sac

Fat

Inferior rectus muscle

The nasolacrimal duct carries tear fluid from the lacrimal sac into the nasal cavity. Fluid leaves the nasolacrimal duct via an opening near the base of the duct.

Nasolacrimal duct

Bone

Nasal cavity

PROTECTING THE EYES

The eye is a delicate structure that needs protection from the many dangers presented by the outside world. The bony brow ridge above each eye and the eye's position fairly deep within its socket help protect the eye from injury. The eyelids, eyelashes, and eyebrows all guard against foreign substances getting into the eye.

In addition, a lubricating film of tear fluid is drawn over the eyeball by the eyelid every time we blink. The final layer of protection is the tough covering of the eyeball itself, made up of the sclera and (at the front of the eye) the transparent cornea.

Protection and movement

Surrounding the eye are various structures that help protect it from harm. Also around the outside of the eye lies a group of muscles that enable the eyeball to swivel in its bony socket.

EYES ON THE MOVE

Thanks to a group of six tiny muscles surrounding them, the eyeballs can turn up and down, from side to side, and even at oblique angles in their sockets. Lacrimal (tear) fluid helps lubricate this movement. Movement of the eyes to look in a particular direction is under voluntary control, but coordination of movement needed for focusing on near and distant objects is automatic and involuntary.

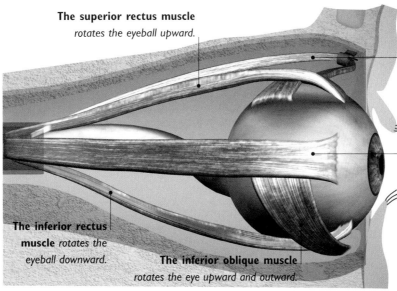

The muscles surrounding the eye *enable it to turn upward, downward, to the left, or to the right.*

Superior rectus

Superior oblique

Lateral rectus

Medial rectus

Inferior oblique

Inferior rectus

The superior rectus muscle *rotates the eyeball upward.*

The superior oblique muscle *rotates the eyeball downward and outward.*

Each muscle *extends from the eyeball toward the the rear of the orbital cavity.*

The lateral rectus muscle *rotates the eye outward. On the other side of the eye, opposite this muscle, lies the medial rectus muscle (see above), which rotates the eyeball inward.*

The inferior rectus muscle *rotates the eyeball downward.*

The inferior oblique muscle *rotates the eye upward and outward.*

WHY IT ALL ENDS IN TEARS

Tears contain mucus to lubricate the eye, the chemical lysozyme to prevent infection, and antibodies that also fight infection. Tear fluid is constantly produced by the lacrimal glands, situated above and behind each eye, to keep the eyeball lubricated. Tears are also triggered by

- **A foreign body** in the eye, such as grit. The body attempts to flush away the irritant with tears.
- **A response to pain** elsewhere in the body. This is an automatic involuntary reflex.

- An outburst of extreme emotion—grief, anger, fear, or happiness—no one has yet worked out why.

From each lacrimal gland, tears travel to the surface of the eye, where much of the fluid evaporates. Excess fluid passes through the openings in the inner corner of the eye (the lacrimal puncta) into the lacrimal sac and then into the nasolacrimal duct and the nasal cavity. This is why the more you cry, the more you need to blow your nose. When tears are coming faster than the lacrimal puncta can cope with them, they overflow down the cheeks.

Getting things in focus

When light rays hit the eye, they are parallel. As they pass through the layers that make up the eye, they become bent (refracted) so that they converge at a spot on the back of the retina. The result is a sharp, clear image.

LOOKING AT SOMETHING IN THE DISTANCE

With the eyes at rest (that is, not attempting to see a close object) the refractive powers of the eye are sufficient to focus the parallel rays of light from a distant object onto the retina so that this object can be seen in sharp focus.

FOCUSING ON A CLOSER OBJECT

When you focus on objects less than about 20 feet away, light rays entering the eye need to bend to a greater degree than they would otherwise. The processes that allow this are called accommodation, convergence, and pupillary constriction.

- **Accommodation** The lens in the eye thickens in order to increase its refractive power.

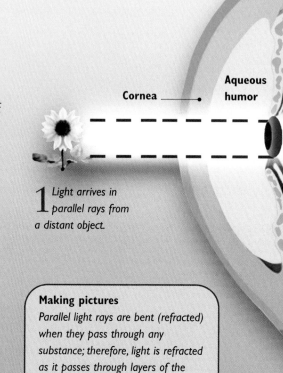

Vitreous humor

Cornea — **Aqueous humor** **Lens**

1 *Light arrives in parallel rays from a distant object.*

2 *The eye's lens bends the light rays inward, causing them to converge on a spot called the fovea centralis, which is within the macula lutea on the retina.*

Making pictures

Parallel light rays are bent (refracted) when they pass through any substance; therefore, light is refracted as it passes through layers of the eye. Unlike the other layers of the eye, the lens has the ability to change its shape and thus alter the degree to which it refracts light.

WHAT HAPPENS WHEN THINGS GO WRONG?

Sometimes parallel rays of light are not brought to a focus on the retina when the eyes are at rest—that is, looking at something in the distance. If sharp sight is to be achieved, an extra glass or plastic lens must be used to change the angle of the light rays before they enter the eye.

Nearsightedness (myopia)

This condition is caused by light rays converging before they reach the retina when accommodation is relaxed. This means that when the eyes are at rest, distant objects are seen as blurred. Accommodation allows someone who is nearsighted to see close objects clearly.

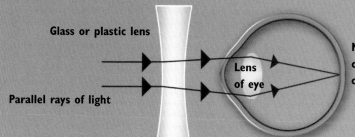

Nearsightedness caused by the eyeball being longer than normal

Glass or plastic lens

Lens of eye

Nearsightedness corrected by a concave lens

Parallel rays of light

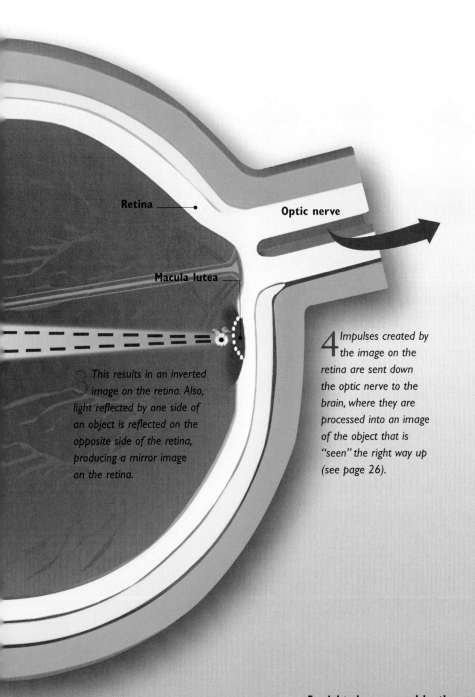

Retina

Optic nerve

Macula lutea

3 This results in an inverted image on the retina. Also, light reflected by one side of an object is reflected on the opposite side of the retina, producing a mirror image on the retina.

4 Impulses created by the image on the retina are sent down the optic nerve to the brain, where they are processed into an image of the object that is "seen" the right way up (see page 26).

- **Convergence** Light rays from an object must focus on the same part of the retina in both eyes to produce a single clear image. When viewing close objects, the eyes swivel inward to ensure that the rays still fall on the same spots. This is known as convergence, and it makes us cross-eyed when we try to focus on objects that are very close to us.
- **Pupillary constriction** When we look at close objects, our pupils shrink to block out the outer rays of light and allow in only those rays that will pass through the central part of the lens. This helps the eye produce a sharp image. The pupil shrinks as a result of the contraction of circular muscles in the iris.

Presbyopia

As people age, the accommodation ability of their eyes decreases so that they no longer see objects that are close as clearly as they once could. They then need glasses with convex lenses for reading and other close work.

Farsightedness (hypermetropia)

This condition occurs when light rays have not converged when they reach the retina. Accommodation naturally corrects slight farsightedness, so distance and near vision are good, but accommodation can't correct severe farsightedness completely, making near vision more blurred than distance vision.

Farsightedness caused by the eyeball being shorter in length than normal

Farsightedness corrected by a convex lens

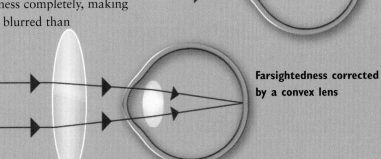

> **Astigmatism**
> Astigmatism is a condition caused by a slight distortion in the shape of the front surface of the eye—the lens or cornea is egg-shaped rather than spherical. This means that not all the parallel rays of light are brought to a point on the retina. It can accompany near-sightedness or farsightedness.

Seeing colors, light, and dark

*We can recognize a vast array of colors and shades thanks
to the millions of specialized light-sensitive cells called rods
and cones, which are located in the retina—the membrane
that lines the eye's interior.*

DIFFERENT COLORS, DIFFERENT WAVELENGTHS

Light rays are somewhere in the middle of the electromagnetic spectrum
(which comprises rays of various wavelengths, from very short wavelengths,
such as X-rays, to very long wavelengths, such as radio waves). Light rays
are the ones detected by the receptors of the eyes.

   The light rays are of different colors depending on their
wavelengths. For example, red is produced by rays with
a long wavelength. Any object that reflects these light
rays and absorbs the others will appear red to us.
Objects that reflect rays of all wavelengths
appear white; those that absorb all
wavelengths appear black. Some objects
reflect different wavelengths to varying
degrees, allowing us to see various
shades of color. You take this
information in via your eyes, but
it is the brain that completes the
process of enabling you to see
such a variety of colors.

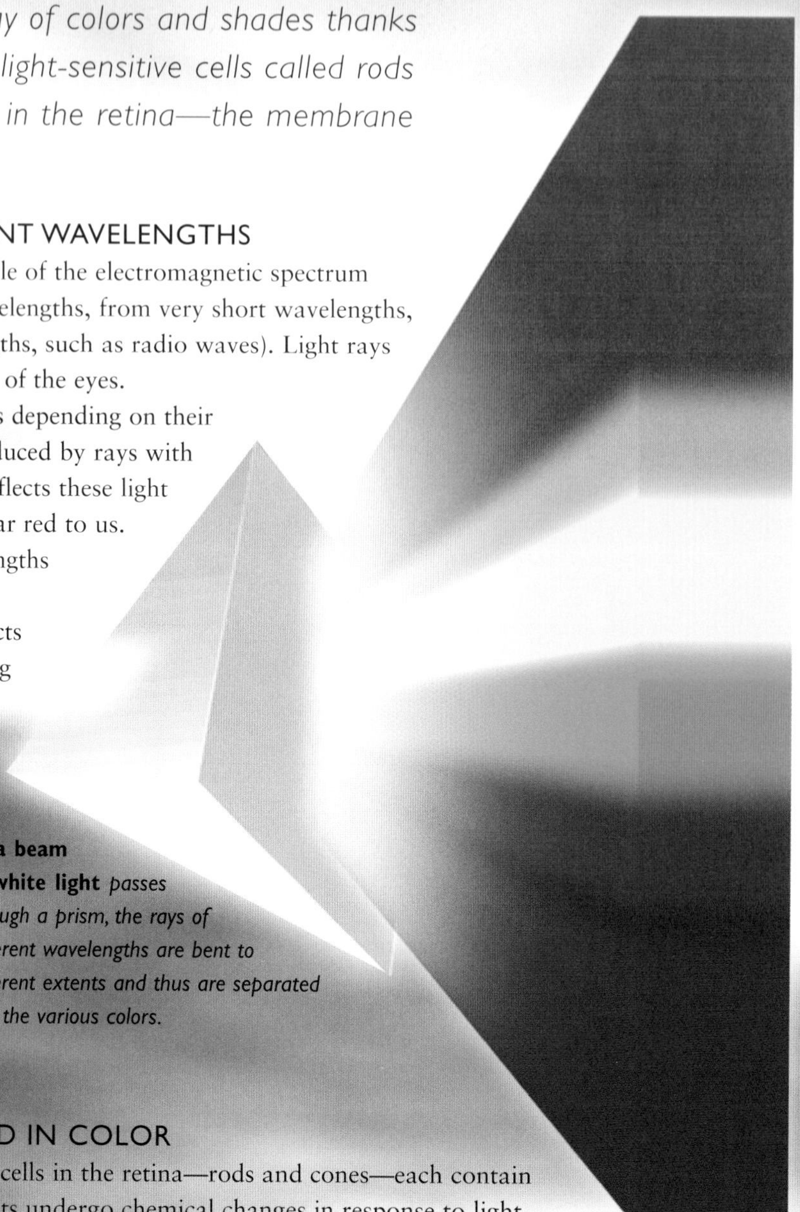

**As a beam
of white light** *passes
through a prism, the rays of
different wavelengths are bent to
different extents and thus are separated
into the various colors.*

Red *has
the longest
wavelength.*

Orange

Yellow

Green

Blue

Indigo

Violet *has
the shortest
wavelength.*

SEEING THE DAYLIGHT WORLD IN COLOR

The two kinds of light-sensitive nerve cells in the retina—rods and cones—each contain
light-sensitive pigments. These pigments undergo chemical changes in response to light,
changes that trigger nerve impulses that pass to the brain for processing. Cones are
activated by bright light. There are three types, each containing a pigment that is
sensitive to either red, blue, or green. They are stimulated to varying degrees to
produce other colors, such as yellow and purple.

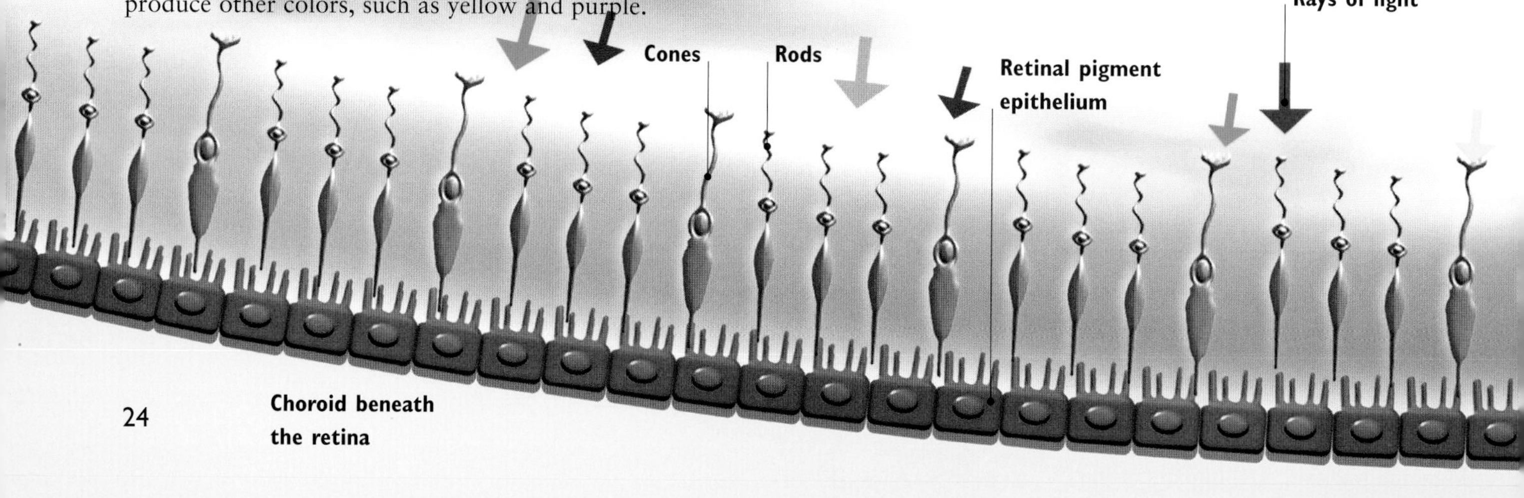

Cones

Rods

**Retinal pigment
epithelium**

Rays of light

**Choroid beneath
the retina**

SEEING THE NIGHTTIME WORLD IN BLACK AND WHITE

Rods contain one pigment only. They are responsible for black and white vision in semidarkness and need only a small amount of light to be activated. This is why you see your surroundings more in black and white than in color when you are in semidarkness.

Adjusting between light and dark

In bright light, cones do all the work, you can see things clearly and in full color, and the pigment in the rods is broken down rapidly. If you move from bright light into a darkened environment, it takes a little while for your eyes to grow accustomed to the darkness so you can see. This is because you must wait for rod pigment to be regenerated so that the rods can take over.

   The pupils also change in response to light and darkness, constricting in bright light to limit the amount of light that can enter the eye and then dilating when the light is dim to allow as much light as possible into the eye.

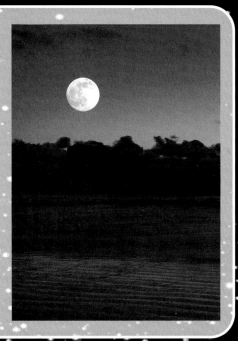

RODS AND CONES

This magnified image from a scanning electron microscope shows rods and cones on the surface of the retina; the cones are wider and more rounded than the rods. They are kept in good condition by the retinal pigment epithelium that lies below them. There are more cones in some parts of the retina than in others. Both rods and cones are connected to other nerve cells, which transmit the nerve impulses generated by rays of light toward the brain, their final destination. There are about 100 million rods and 7 million cones in the retina of each eye.

The journey from eye to brain

The vast amount of information taken in by the eyes in the form of light rays would mean nothing to us without the brain to process them. Nerve impulses are sent through a system of pathways to the occipital lobe at the back of the brain.

The optic tracts *are the pathways of the optic nerves between the optic chiasma and the brain.*

MAKING THE CONNECTION

Nerve impulses leave the eyes via the two optic nerves, which meet at the optic chiasma in the brain. Nerve fibers from the inner side of each retina cross over here so that each side of the brain receives information from both eyes. Half the information from each eye is sent to each side of the brain. The nerve impulses then continue their journey. Many impulses are transmitted to the visual cortex of the occipital lobe, at the back of the cerebrum. Some are sent to the cerebellum, at the base of the brain, where they are integrated with information from the ears, muscles, and joints to maintain balance and help in movement.

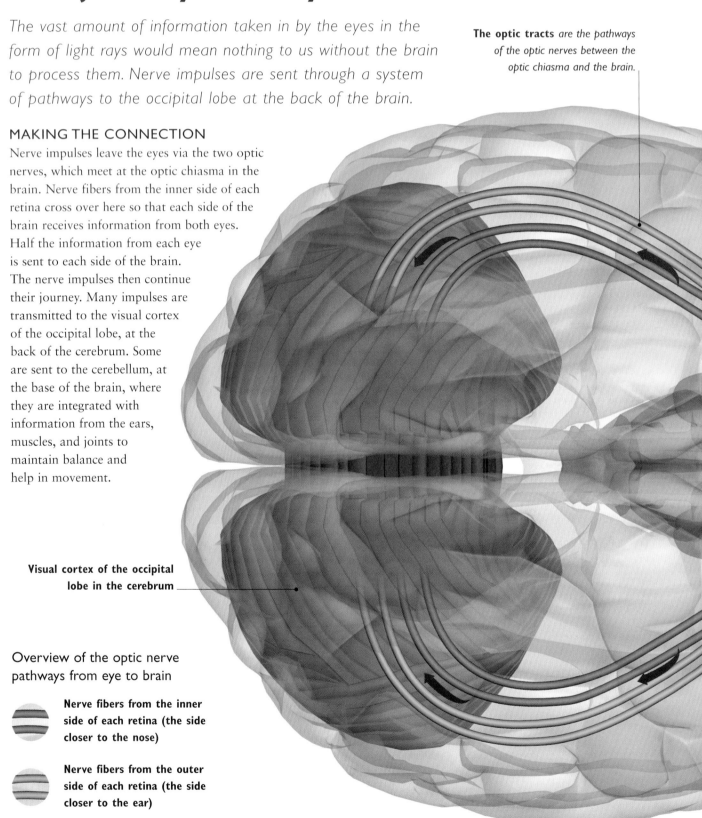

Visual cortex of the occipital lobe in the cerebrum

Overview of the optic nerve pathways from eye to brain

Nerve fibers from the inner side of each retina (the side closer to the nose)

Nerve fibers from the outer side of each retina (the side closer to the ear)

Everyone has a dominant eye that he or she uses more than the other. Your dominant eye is the one you use when looking into the viewfinder of a camera or threading a needle.

Side view of the eye and brain

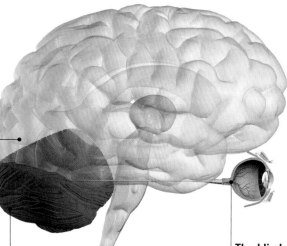

The occipital lobe *is where information from the eye in the form of nerve impulses is processed into visual images that we can understand.*

The optic nerves *are made up of nerve fibers that receive information from the rods and cones in the retina.*

The eye viewed from overhead

The cerebellum *combines information from the eyes, ears, and muscles to ensure that the body's movements are smooth and coordinated. It also plays a key role in maintaining balance and posture.*

The blind spot (optic disk) *is the point where the optic nerve leaves the eye.*

The optic chiasma *is where the nerve impulses from both eyes meet.*

THE BLIND SPOT
The optic disk is the area on the back of the eye where the optic nerve leaves the eye carrying sensory information to be processed by the brain. It is often called the blind spot because there are no light-sensitive cells in this area, so it does not register light; as a result, it causes a blind spot in the visual field.

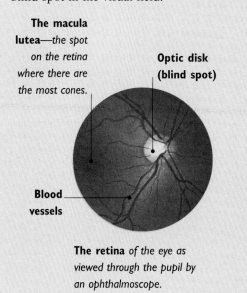

The macula lutea—*the spot on the retina where there are the most cones.*

Optic disk (blind spot)

Blood vessels

The retina of the eye as viewed through the pupil by an ophthalmoscope.

Inside the mouth

The mouth is not simply the entry point for food and air; its ingenious structure allows it to fulfill several other functions, including forming food into a bolus (ball) ready to be swallowed, tasting different flavors, and helping form sounds.

EXPLORING THE MOUTH

The cavity of the mouth is bordered by the lips at the front, the cheeks at the sides, the palate above, and the tongue below. The tongue is essentially a muscle. It is made up of a body (the part that you can see) and a root attached by muscles to the hyoid bone in the neck. In the mouth lie the teeth, resilient structures that break down food to make it ready to begin the digestive process.

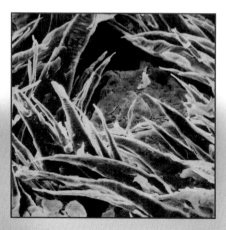

The surface of the tongue
The upper surface of the tongue is covered with tiny projections called papillae. In this false-color scanning electron micrograph, filiform papillae (pink) surround a fungiform papillae (yellow).

The hard palate is the bony front part of the roof of the mouth.

The soft palate is the back part of the roof of the mouth.

The uvula lies at the back of the soft palate. It is an extension of the soft palate.

The tonsils are swellings toward the back of the mouth. Together with the adenoids, they form a ring around the entrance to the pharynx. They produce cells called lymphocytes, which attack infective organisms as they enter the body, thus forming one of the body's first lines of defense.

The tongue lies in the floor of the mouth. It moves food around the mouth so that it can be broken down by the teeth and then forms it into a bolus (ball) to be swallowed. The tongue is also the site of thousands of taste buds that allow us to detect many different flavors and of sensory receptors that detect touch, temperature, and pain.

The teeth are made of materials hard enough to cut and chew food; they are set in softer gums that provide a seal around the neck of the tooth to prevent bacteria from attacking the underlying bone.

PREPARING FOOD TO BE SWALLOWED

Food is moved around the mouth by the tongue and the muscles of the cheeks. It is chewed by the teeth and mixed with saliva, which is stimulated by taste and the action of chewing. This turns the food into a softened mass, which the tongue shapes into a bolus and pushes to the back of the mouth, ready to be swallowed. The muscles of the pharynx push the bolus into the esophagus, which propels the food down its length to the stomach.

TAKING IN AIR

The mouth has close connections with the nose and the upper part of the respiratory system, all by way of the pharynx. This passageway extends from the back of the mouth, up behind the nose, and down to the esophagus. Air gets into the lungs via the larynx, which extends from the pharynx and down into the trachea (the windpipe).

SPEECH

The mouth plays a key role in communication. Sounds produced by air passing through the vocal cords in the larynx are shaped into speech, song, and other sounds by the mouth, tongue, and lips.

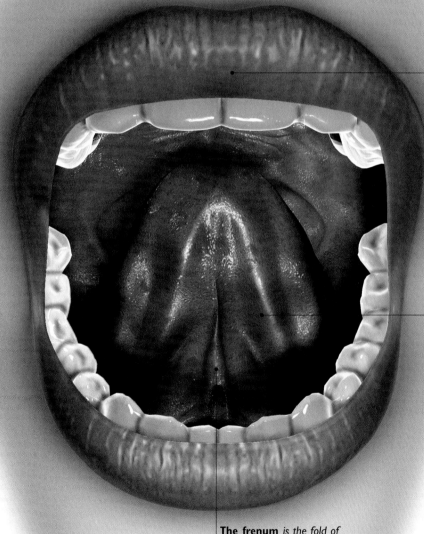

The alveolar ridge *is the bony structure behind the upper front teeth. It plays an important role in speech – key sounds such as "t" and "n" are produced when the tongue touches the alveolar ridge.*

The lower side of the tongue *has a surface that is thinner and more delicate than that of the tongue's upper side.*

The frenum *is the fold of mucous membrane that runs down the center of the underside of the tongue.*

The lips and tongue have so many touch receptors that they are among the most sensitive parts of the body.

Teeth

Before the process of digestion can begin, food must be broken down into smaller pieces. This is the function of the teeth, which cut food and then grind it down. The teeth are helped in their work by the tongue, which moves the food around the mouth.

Tooth enamel is the hardest substance in the human body.

GAINING A FULL SET

Everyone has two sets of teeth in his or her lifetime: the deciduous (baby or milk) teeth and the permanent teeth. The complete set of 32 permanent teeth is usually present by the early 20s. There are 20 deciduous teeth, which begin to appear when babies are about 6 months old. They are all present by around 2 years of age. Replacement of deciduous teeth by permanent teeth begins at about 6 years old. The roots of the deciduous teeth are slowly reabsorbed when permanent teeth start to push through above them.

SHAPING UP

The teeth are embedded in bone. There are four different shapes for the different functions required, but all teeth have the same basic structure. The incisors and canines, at the front, are more pointed and are used for cutting food, whereas the premolar and molar teeth grind food to allow it to be mixed thoroughly with saliva before it is swallowed.

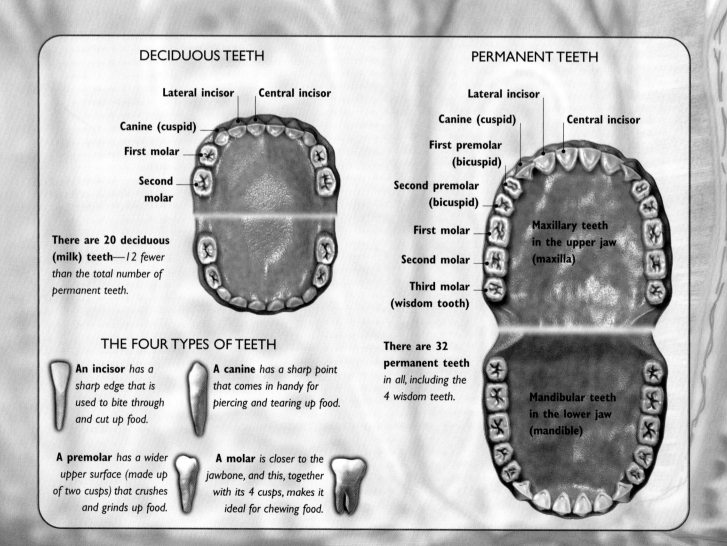

DECIDUOUS TEETH

Lateral incisor Central incisor
Canine (cuspid)
First molar
Second molar

There are 20 deciduous (milk) teeth—*12 fewer than the total number of permanent teeth.*

PERMANENT TEETH

Lateral incisor
Canine (cuspid)   Central incisor
First premolar (bicuspid)
Second premolar (bicuspid)
First molar
Second molar
Third molar (wisdom tooth)

Maxillary teeth in the upper jaw (maxilla)

Mandibular teeth in the lower jaw (mandible)

There are 32 permanent teeth *in all, including the 4 wisdom teeth.*

THE FOUR TYPES OF TEETH

An incisor *has a sharp edge that is used to bite through and cut up food.*

A canine *has a sharp point that comes in handy for piercing and tearing up food.*

A premolar *has a wider upper surface (made up of two cusps) that crushes and grinds up food.*

A molar *is closer to the jawbone, and this, together with its 4 cusps, makes it ideal for chewing food.*

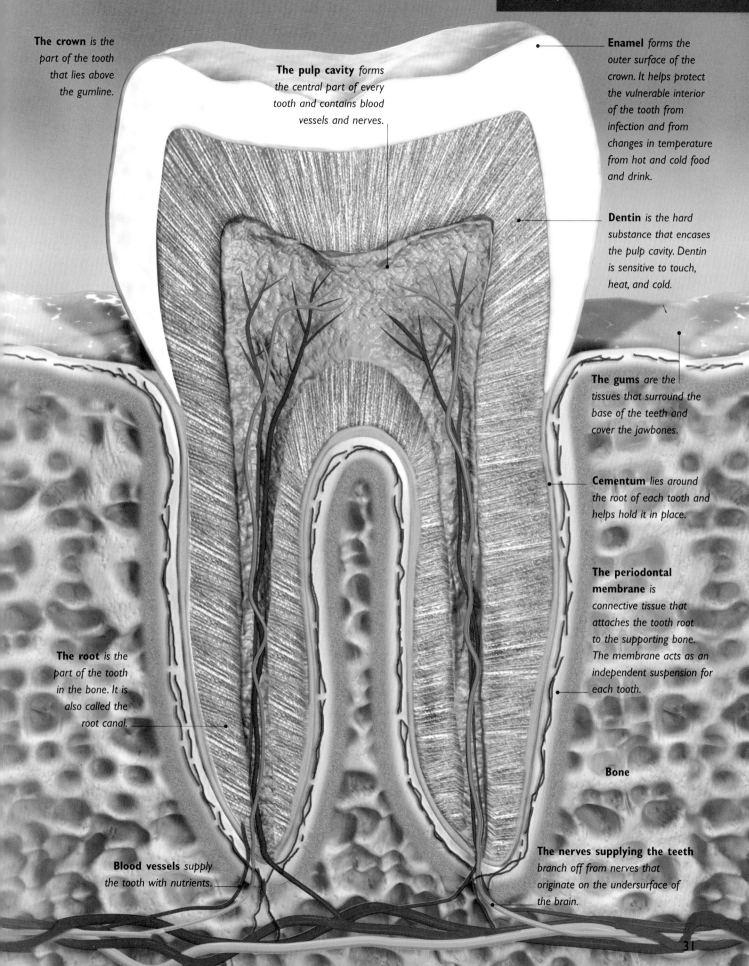

The crown *is the part of the tooth that lies above the gumline.*

The pulp cavity *forms the central part of every tooth and contains blood vessels and nerves.*

Enamel *forms the outer surface of the crown. It helps protect the vulnerable interior of the tooth from infection and from changes in temperature from hot and cold food and drink.*

Dentin *is the hard substance that encases the pulp cavity. Dentin is sensitive to touch, heat, and cold.*

The gums *are the tissues that surround the base of the teeth and cover the jawbones.*

Cementum *lies around the root of each tooth and helps hold it in place.*

The periodontal membrane *is connective tissue that attaches the tooth root to the supporting bone. The membrane acts as an independent suspension for each tooth.*

Bone

The root *is the part of the tooth in the bone. It is also called the root canal.*

Blood vessels *supply the tooth with nutrients.*

The nerves supplying the teeth *branch off from nerves that originate on the undersurface of the brain.*

Taste and saliva

Two important processes that take place in the mouth are taste and the release of saliva, which helps kick-start the digestive process. Different tastes are detected primarily by the tongue.

The salivary glands produce between 1 and 1.5 quarts of saliva every single day.

WHAT IS SALIVA AND WHAT DOES IT DO?

Saliva is produced by three pairs of salivary glands and passes through ducts into the mouth, where it is joined by mucus from many small glands in the mouth lining. The resulting mix of saliva and mucus (generally referred to simply as "saliva") is almost entirely water but also contains the enzymes salivary amylase and lysozyme, plus antibodies and mineral salts. Saliva has a number of functions.

- It lubricates the mouth and food so food can be moved around easily and formed into a bolus to be swallowed.
- It contributes to the taste sensation—food has to be mixed with saliva before it can stimulate the taste buds.
- Amylase in saliva begins to break down starches.
- The antibodies and lysozyme in saliva form part of the body's defenses against infection.
- Its mineral salts help protect the teeth from acid.

Saliva is produced continuously and also as an automatic response to the sight, smell, or even thought of food.

The parotid glands *open into the mouth near the second upper molar.*

The submandibular glands *open onto the floor of the mouth.*

The sublingual glands *open onto the floor of the mouth in front of the submandibular glands.*

The salivary glands *are made up of lobules lined with secretory cells. Tiny ducts from the secretory cells carry the saliva into larger ducts that drain into the mouth.*

Circumvallate papillae *are the largest of the papillae and are circular in shape. A circumvallate papilla can be associated with up to 100 taste buds.*

Fungiform papillae *are most numerous along the edges and tip of the tongue. They are mushroom-shaped, as their name indicates. Each one has about five taste buds.*

Filiform papillae *are the smallest of the papillae and are scattered over the front two thirds of the tongue. They are threadlike and are not associated with taste buds.*

The center of the tongue *does not have many taste receptors*

Bitter

Sour

Salty

Sweet

TASTE AND THE TONGUE

Papillae are the tiny projections on the upper surface of the tongue. Along the sides of the particular papillae known as circumvallate and fungiform lie special nerve endings called taste buds. These nerve endings terminate in tiny hairs that project from the tongue's surface and detect different tastes. The nerve impulses generated are transported to the brain.

Different tastes are detected in separate parts of the tongue. For example, bitterness is detected at the back and sweetness at the front. Some taste buds are also found in the lining of the soft palate and the pharynx. The work of the taste buds is complemented by the sensation of smell, which plays an important role in the detection of tastes.

A TASTE BUD

Taste buds *are found around the edges of circumvallate and fungiform papillae. Each taste bud contains about 40 gustatory cells that send nerve impulses to the thalamus, in the brain.*

Gustatory hairs—*these microvilli (tiny hairs) act as sensory receptors when bathed in saliva.*

A pore, *sometimes called a taste pore, on the surface of the tongue.*

Epithelial cells *make up the outermost layer—the epithelium—of the tongue.*

Supporting cells *separate the gustatory cells from each other and from the epithelium.*

Gustatory cells, *also called taste cells, are the specialized receptor cells that transmit nerve impulses from the gustatory hairs to the nerve fibers.*

Nerve fibers *transmit impulses from the gustatory cells to the thalamus, in the brain.*

The mouth and speech

Sound is produced in the larynx and then shaped by the different parts of the mouth. The tongue, lips, teeth, jaw, and soft palate all help to form the sounds that make up words by controlling airflow through the mouth.

PRODUCING SOUND

Most speech sounds originate with air being expelled from the lungs. Air travels from the lungs to the trachea (windpipe) and then to the larynx (voice box), where the vocal cords are found. As air passes through them, the vocal cords vibrate, which causes the air to resonate. When you begin to speak, the vocal cords vibrate enough to produce a buzzing sound. Not all speech sounds require the vocal cords to vibrate in this way; for example, the sound "zzz" does but "sss" does not.

HOW YOUR MOUTH SHAPES SOUND

Having passed through the larynx, the air moves into the pharynx and either travels through the throat into the mouth or behind the soft palate and into the nasal cavity. In order to form words, you modify the sound of the resonating air by altering the shape of the cavities through which the air passes. When it comes to shaping sound in the mouth, the tongue, jaw, soft palate, lips, and teeth are all important, and related structures also have roles to play.

Vowel sounds

Vowel sounds are generated when air is able to travel unimpeded through the open mouth. The individual vowel sounds are produced by changing the shape and size of the cavities that the air passes through. The lips and tongue are of particular significance: Compare the difference in lip position, for example, when pronouncing the sounds "oo" and "ee."

Consonants

Consonants are produced when a barrier is put in the way of the airflow. For example,
- **Narrowing the passage** through which the air flows creates friction in the moving air that produces sounds such as "sss," "sh," "th," and "f."
- **Stopping the flow** of air produces "t" when using the tip of the tongue, "k" when using the body of the tongue, and "p" when using the lips.
- **Using the soft palate** to force air into the nasal cavity produces "n" and "m."

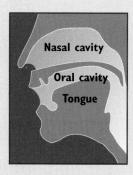 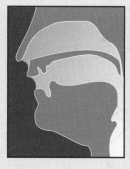 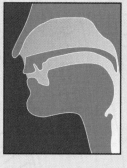 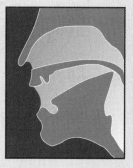 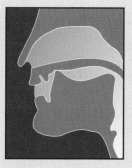

Nasal cavity
Oral cavity
Tongue

Pronouncing "i" as in "hit"
The soft palate is raised and tensed for the "i" sound, and perhaps there is more lip spreading than in "oo" as in food.

Pronouncing "o" as in "book"
The body of the tongue is less raised than in "i" and there is normally more lip rounding.

Pronouncing "p" and "b"
With lips together, air pressure builds up, so that when the lips are opened, sounds called bilabial plosives are heard (bilabial means using both lips). The voiced sound is "b" whereas "p" is voiceless— that is, it does not require the vocal cords to vibrate.

Pronouncing "k" and "g"
The back of the tongue is raised and the air builds behind, so when the tongue releases on these sounds, called velar plosives, a "k" or "g" sound is heard. (Velar means using the soft palate.) "K" is a voiceless sound, whereas "g" is voiced by vocal cord vibration.

Pronouncing "n"
The sound is made like "t" and "d," with the front of the tongue on the alveolar ridge. The soft palate is lowered to allow air to pass into the nasal cavity above to produce a nasal sound. If you pinch your nose when making this sound, the sound will suddenly stop.

The soft palate lowers for nasal sounds such as "m," "n," and "ng" and when we speak softly and warmly. It lifts up when we need to shout or belt out sound such as in singing, contributing to a bright, clear sound.

The teeth are important for making the "sss" sound, which is why this sound often gets distorted in people with missing teeth. Sounds such as "f" and "v" are made by pressing the front teeth onto the lower lip.

How languages differ

All English speech sounds start with air being expelled from the lungs, but this is not the case with some other languages. Glottalic sounds, made by using the glottis (the gap between the vocal cords), can employ air moving inward (implosive sounds) as an alternative to air moving outward (explosive sounds). "Click" sounds, originating with the tongue or lips, are widely used in non-European languages. Pharyngeal sounds are made when the tongue is lowered and retracted, resulting in the walls of the pharynx constricting.

The alveolar ridge behind the upper front teeth is used to make "t," "d," and "n"; the front of the tongue articulates against the ridge. It is also useful for making trill sounds, an ability that not everyone has and that may be genetically determined.

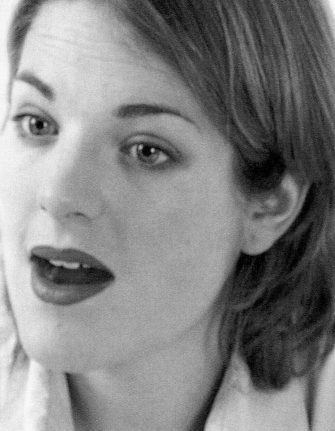

The lips are important for sounds such as "p," "b," and "m." Air builds up behind the closed lips so that when they are opened, we hear these "plosive" sounds. Some people use more lip rounding than others, which gives their speech a "darker" quality. Others use more lip spreading, the extreme being to talk with a broad smile. This makes speech brighter, because sound is resonating in a smaller space than in lip rounding. It is thought that women use a greater range of lip movements than men—if you're a man trying to imitate a woman, this is one of the easiest ways to do it.

The tongue is important for shaping vowel sounds and also contributes to accents. A tongue that is flat in the mouth and pulled toward the back will make speech sound swallowed and duller, whereas if the tongue is high in the mouth and more toward the front, the speech will sound brighter.

The lower jaw is the part that moves in speech. Jaw tension can make speech sound aggressive and may be a result of stress; it can also cause teeth grinding at night. Tension can also lead to mumbling and a held-back voice. A relaxed jaw and open mouth immediately make speech sound clearer, because there is more room to move your tongue and make use of the space in your mouth. Actors and singers have to practice using a loose jaw to get the best out of their voice and articulation.

A day in the life of the eyes and mouth

From the moment you awaken to the moment you go to sleep, your eyes and mouth are hard at work. Your eyes are constantly appraising the world around you, enabling you to react to situations. Your mouth enables you to communicate and takes in the food you need.

TEAMWORK

The eyes "read" a situation, and among the parts of the body that respond is, of course, the mouth. In this interplay between eyes and mouth, the nervous system and brain play essential roles, and other senses—most directly touch and taste but also hearing and smell—are involved as well.

7:00 A.M. Waking up

You look around you as you awaken. It is still half-dark, but you can see thanks to the light-sensitive cells in the retina known as rods, which are stimulated by dim light. You reach out to pull back the curtain, and daylight floods in. At first, the light seems almost blinding, but gradually you grow accustomed to the brightness as the cones, the cells in the retina sensitive to brighter light, take over for the rods. You can now see in color rather than in shades of gray.

12:00 P.M. Lunch time

You pop out to the local deli to buy lunch. You are so hungry that just the thought of food starts your salivary juices flowing by triggering nerve impulses in the salivation center in the brain stem (the base structure of the brain that links it to the spinal cord). As you eat, you can detect various flavors because of the action of taste buds, mainly located on the upper surface of the tongue. A network of nerves carries impulses from these taste receptors to the cerebral cortex of the brain to be processed. The information from the taste buds is complemented by other sensations, in particular smell, which is detected by highly sensitive hairs in the roof of the nasal cavity and also processed in the cortex of the brain. Other receptors in the mouth gauge the temperature of food and drink. Memories of tastes are stored, and the brain tells you which foods you like and which you don't.

A feast for the eyes and mouth
Although the eyes have nothing to do with digestion, they play a big part in stimulating the appetite and choosing what we want to eat. This colorful meal is low in fat, good for diabetics who want to avoid eye problems. Poultry is a good source of zinc, vital to eye health, and the salad and fruit dressing protect against gum disease.

12:00 A.M. Dream on

You close your eyes and go to sleep, but for part of the night your eyes are still active. The electrical activity in your brain varies, producing two main phases of sleep. During REM (rapid eye movement) sleep, the muscles of your body do not move and you lie completely still. However, your eyes are moving rapidly all the time, and your eyelids, although closed, are fluttering. This phase is preceded by a period of non-REM sleep, during which your muscles are relaxed but you can still move around and change position. In REM sleep, brain activity is similar to when we are awake, and it is during these phases that we dream. We pass through both phases up to five times a night. About one quarter of the time asleep is spent in REM sleep.

8:00 P.M. Enjoying a good cry

After work, it's finally time to relax. You go to the movies with a friend. The film has its sad moments, and as the story reaches its climax, your eyes fill with tears. It has not yet been established precisely why strong emotion causes us to cry—why we cry when there is no physical stimulus, such as pain. Because we often feel better after a good cry, however, scientists speculate that tears are triggered by stressful feelings because they are a means of alleviating these feelings. It certainly works—you dry your eyes and emerge from the theater talking about what a good film it was.

3:00 P.M. Communicating

You are involved in a group discussion at work. How do you know how to interact appropriately? Communicating involves more than the production of words by the larynx and mouth. The higher parts of your brain involved in feelings influence how you respond, but in addition, you must be able to understand what you hear and see and to form what you are going to say in your mind. Wernicke's area, in the cerebral cortex (the outer layer of the brain), is responsible for assimilating what you hear so you can understand it. In Broca's area, also in the cerebral cortex, sentences are put together, drawing on the vocabulary and grammar stored in your memory.

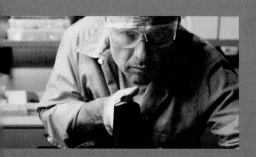 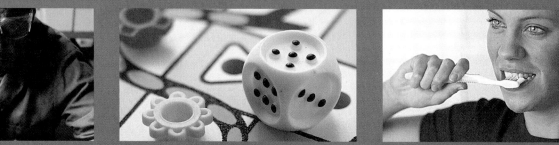 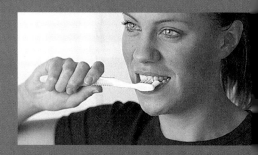

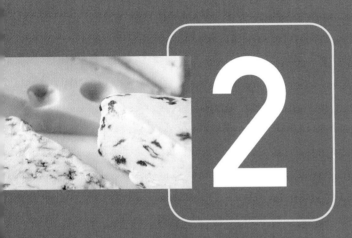

2

Keeping your eyes and mouth healthy

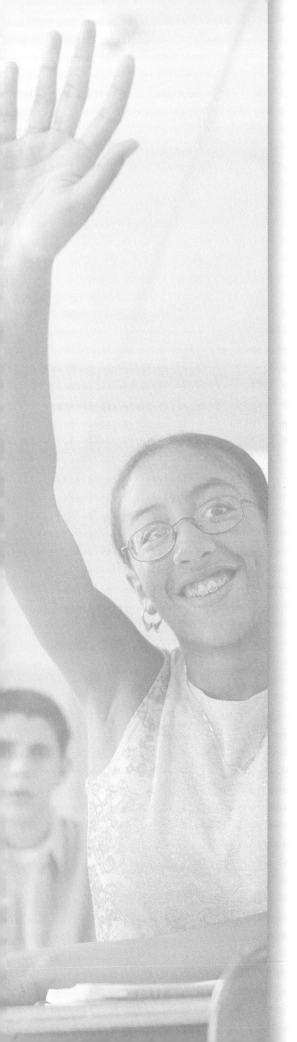

TAKE CHARGE OF YOUR HEALTH

The eyes work best when they are not overloaded and if any problems are addressed promptly with corrective lenses. When it comes to the teeth and oral health, prevention really is better than cure, so adopting good habits early is the smart move.

 41 *The eyes are good at taking care of themselves, but it pays to avoid infection and strain at any age.*

 44 *Eyes are not static; they evolve as we age. Understanding the normal aging process helps identify potential problems early.*

 48 *Deteriorating sight does not have to mean an end to enjoyable activities: There are many coping strategies and resources for those with poor sight.*

 53 *Conventional eye specialists are dubious about the value of eye exercises, although some individuals believe that they work.*

 54 *The teeth and gums change as we age: Understanding the threats to them at different ages is a good first step to oral health.*

 56 *There is a great deal you can do to take care of your teeth from childhood to old age. A daily oral hygiene routine is not difficult to devise.*

Take care of your eyes

Delicate yet robust, with their own protective mechanisms, the eyes need little in the way of extra care under most circumstances. However, it makes sense to know how to best take care of one of your body's major assets.

Most people would probably rate the ability to see as one of the most important of their five senses. It is vital that sight problems be picked up early and treated effectively, so regular eye tests from infancy on are a must. An undiagnosed or untreated problem can lead to unnecessary permanent damage. Day to day, we can help our eyes avoid strain and keep free of infection by introducing as few foreign bodies into the eye area as possible.

HOW EYES TAKE CARE OF THEMSELVES

Our eyes have their own highly effective hygiene system to deal with dirt, bacteria, and other materials that affect the eye daily. The mainstay of this system are tears, made of a remarkable fluid that acts as a cleansing solution, has a powerful bactericidal action, contributes to immune defense, and provides nutrition and oxygen to the eyes, all at the same time. The eyelids and tear fluid work together as a windshield wiper-and-washer system: The lids smear tear fluid over the clear screen that is the cornea.

HOW TO HELP OUR EYES

It is important to remember that the outside of the eye is as delicate as the inside of the body, and it should be treated with due care. That said, the natural eye hygiene system needs little assistance in addition to daily face washing.

No need to meddle

For anyone with normal, healthy eyes, commercial eye hygiene preparations are not necessary but are harmless as long as they are not out of date. However, homemade preparations for soothing eyes (such as chamomile rinses) are not risk-free. If left sitting for any length of time, these can turn into bacterial soup. All in all, the eyes are best left alone.

Special treatment for babies

Babies' tears are more dilute than those of an adult, so babies' eyes are more prone to infection. They can also have tear flow problems, caused by blockage of the drainage duct by the side of the nose, producing crusting around the eyes. This needs to be removed by gentle washing.

GUARD AGAINST INFECTION

Makeup, contact lenses, and fingers can all harm the eyes. Problems arise most frequently when the delicate

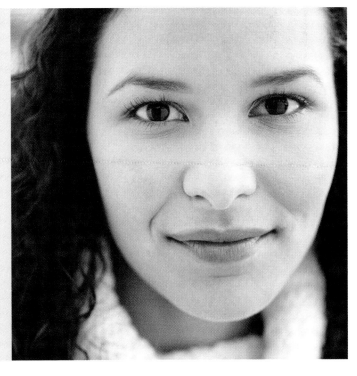

THE EYES AS COMMUNICATORS

We not only see with our eyes, we communicate with them as well. In fact, a message from the eyes is so powerful that prolonged eye contact is rare, except when two people are caught up by the extreme emotions of anger or love. As "windows to the soul," the eyes can give away our innermost feelings, to the extent that people will sometimes wear sunglasses to limit their nonverbal communication with others. Some of the ways eyes give away our thoughts and feelings include the following:

- **Pupil dilation** induced by a surge of adrenaline indicates surprise, especially if accompanied by raising the eyebrows.
- **Increased blink rate** is associated with nervousness.
- **Raising the upper lids** is a sign of fear; if the inner eyebrow also dips down, it is a sign of anger.

cornea at the front of the eye is damaged or when particles of foreign matter gain entry to the eye.

Care with contacts

Contact lenses are valuable visual aids that are of great benefit to the vast majority of users but a problem for a few. Essentially, lenses are foreign bodies that can carry infection to the eye if basic hygiene rules are relaxed. Soft contacts have a worse reputation for this than hard ones. The safety rules are simple:

- Always wash your hands before handling your lenses.
- Follow cleaning procedures to the letter.

Is bathing the eyes ever a good idea?

It is never necessary to bathe eyes that are healthy and not too dry: not in tap water, distilled water, a commercial preparation, or a homemade solution. In fact, bathing healthy eyes can be harmful, because you may actually introduce an infection into the eye.

If a foreign body gets into the eye—grit for instance—the standard first-aid procedure is to wash out the foreign particles with sterile water. For eyes in need of medication, eye drops are normally prescribed. To soften eye crusts or a stye, a solution held in an eye bath may be gently wiped across the affected area, as long as a clean cotton swab is used with each wipe and the used swab is never returned to the eye bath.

ASK THE EXPERT

- Always use fresh storage solution.
- Keep the storage case clean. Use contact lens multipurpose or soaking solution.
- Don't be tempted to use tap water to clean lenses or the storage case. Tap water contains an infectious organism called Acanthamoeba, which has caused corneal ulcers in a few contact lens wearers.
- Never use saliva to moisten lenses.
- Take out contact lenses before swimming or wear goggles as well.
- Do not reuse disposable lenses— this is very risky.
- Sleeping in day-wear lenses greatly increases the chance of infection.

The hazards of eye makeup

- An accidental poke in the eye with a mascara brush or eyeliner pencil can damage the cornea and trigger an infection.
- Spitting in eye makeup to soften it is an obvious bacterial hazard, as is sharing makeup with others.
- Using out-of-date products carries the risk that the eye makeup no longer has effective preservatives.

HAVE REGULAR EYE CHECKS

It is sometimes believed, wrongly, that it is difficult to test children's eyes before they can read. Babies and children can be tested using a variety of toys and games; being unable to read is no obstacle to a sight test.

A good time for a first test is at about a year old, followed by another at roughly 18 months, and then at 3 years. This will allow any problems to be picked up promptly, before a child starts school. It is also usually easier for younger children to accept wearing glasses: Older children, who are already at school, may be more reluctant to wear them.

Experts recommend an eye test every year for schoolchildren. A child's vision is fully developed by the age of 8, when a problem such as squint or lazy eye may become permanent if it has been left untreated until this time.

Adult eyes should be tested every 2 years as a minimum and ideally every year, especially for anyone who drives, who already wears corrective lenses, or whose work involves using a computer or video screen.

AVOID EYE STRAIN

Eye strain is generally caused by focusing for too long on a fixed object when the surrounding lighting is poor. The condition can be triggered by activities such as reading, watching television, or working at a computer screen.

The symptoms are unpleasant and debilitating. They can include a frontal headache, blurred vision, and eyes that may be dry and scratchy or too watery. Sometimes there may be a temporary sensation of near-sightedness, but this clears rapidly after work at the computer has finished. Eye strain does not cause the sufferer's eyesight to deteriorate permanently.

To stop eye strain, you need to remove the cause. Simple ways of doing this include

- improving lighting;
- removing any problems with glare that you might be experiencing; and
- taking short breaks at regular intervals from the activity that is causing the eye strain.

In addition, if you are suffering from eye strain, it is best to get an optometrist to check whether there is any underlying problem with focusing or any other eye disorder.

CHOOSING EYEGLASSES

Eyeglasses come in a tremendous range of styles. Your choice of frame will be influenced to an extent by your prescription (stronger lenses tend to look better in smaller frames), but a few general guidelines should help you find a flattering style. The frame should reach no higher than the line of your eyebrows and be no wider than the width of your face at the temples. Certain frames tend to suit certain face shapes, of which there are six: square, round, oval, long, triangular, and heart-shaped.

Frames can also be chosen to enhance or play down certain facial features:

- A low-set bridge seems to shorten a long nose.
- A high-set bridge, in line with the top of the frame, plays down a short nose.
- A thin or clear bridge appears to add width between close-set eyes.
- A colored bridge makes eyes seem closer together.

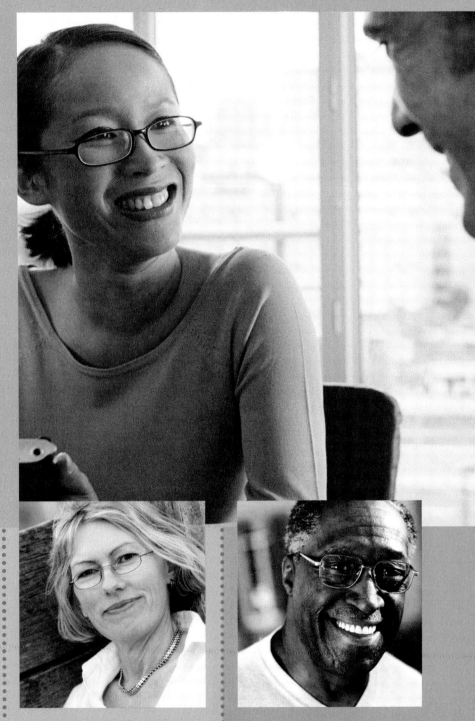

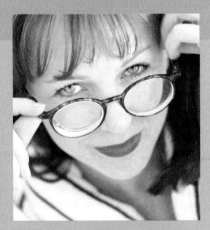

Let frames compliment hair color
If you have auburn hair, consider warm colors in brown, gold, copper, or bronze. If you have darker hair and eyes, consider a rich, deep color for your frames (as shown top right).

A harmonious balance works best
With fair or gray hair and pale skin, lightweight styles in delicate colors often provide the best balance. Bold colors can make a strong, flattering style statement but may be a mistake unless chosen carefully.

Simplicity wins every time
If you have very dark skin, metal frames in simple shapes and colors may suit you better than brightly colored plastic frames, pastels, or very dark colors.

How eyes change with age

The eyes alter in strength from infancy on. Vision sharpens after a "blurry" start at birth, but eyes begin to lose power in early middle age, and the risk of eye illness increases as we grow older.

A BABY'S EYES

A common misconception is that newborn babies can't see. Certainly their sight is poor, although they do have some close vision and can make out their mother's face when it is close. But a lot still needs to be done to improve the interaction between retina and brain and to see clearly.

Babies begin to learn to focus between 1 and 2 months old, by which time they can track a moving object, particularly one they like, such as a face or a shiny rattle. The extraocular muscles are beginning to coordinate, although the tracking will be rather erratic for a few more months. Depth perception is in place by 4 months old, so by that time a baby can grab things more effectively. Color vision is present from around birth but babies appreciate only primary colors; they need until about 9 months old to notice other colors and to incorporate the various tones and hues. Color vision continues to become more refined after this time, as does distance vision. By 9 months old, an infant's vision is almost as acute as an adult's.

Retinopathy of prematurity

Babies born prematurely, when the lungs are still underdeveloped and therefore in need of oxygen from an incubator, are at risk of a condition called "retinopathy of prematurity" (ROP). This occurs because the high oxygen levels necessary for survival can turn out to be toxic to the developing blood vessels in the retina; the abnormal blood vessels leak, and, in severe cases, there is retinal scarring. An ophthalmologist can treat the abnormal retinal tissue of these severe cases with laser or cryotherapy to halt the progression towards blindness. However, about 1 percent of premature babies are blinded by ROP, and much higher numbers will have some visual failing. Babies born before 28 weeks and with a birth weight of less than 2 pounds, 11 ounces are most at risk because their newly forming retinal vessels are particularly vulnerable.

CHILDHOOD EYE DISORDERS

During the complex process of eye and brain development that results in vision, there are lots of things that can and do go wrong. These events create the common eye disorders squint, "lazy eye," and nystagmus.

According to the National PTA, more than 10 million children age 10 and under have vision problems. These are often undetected and misdiagnosed as learning disorders.

Squint and lazy eye

Strabismus, or squint (see page 145), is a condition in which an eye turns away from the object being viewed so that both eyes do not work together. Squint can develop in adults, but it is particularly associated with children: It is present in about 4 percent of all children and is screened for in preschool checkups. Squinting eyes can turn in toward the nose (esotropia) or out away from the nose (exotropia), and the squint can be there all the time (constant squint) or only some of the time (intermittent squint).

When the eyes are not working together, binocular vision is lost and the brain can no longer fuse the images from both eyes into one stereoscopic image. In such a situation, the child may have double vision, and when the squint is

---

IT'S NOT TRUE!

"20/20 vision equals perfect vision"

The term 20/20 vision refers to the sharpness with which an object or scene is viewed from a distance of 20 feet: A person with 20/20 vision can see clearly what should normally be seen at that distance. Someone with 20/80 vision, in contrast, can only see what a person with normal sight can register clearly at 80 feet from a distance of 20 feet. However, 20/20 vision is not perfect vision, simply because there are so many factors in addition to clarity that contribute to good vision. These include depth perception, the ability to focus on close objects, color vision, peripheral vision, and eye coordination.

constant, the brain overcomes the double vision by suppressing the sight in the weaker, squinting eye. If the suppression of vision is allowed to continue, the visual loss may become permanent. Medically, the condition is called amblyopia but it is known more commonly as "lazy eye."

Treatment is directed toward getting both eyes back into alignment and the best sight possible out of the weaker eye to achieve fused binocular vision. It is not true that if left alone children will outgrow squint. They need medical intervention, which can involve glasses, an eye patch, and eye exercises, and the earlier treatment can start, the better the final outcome is likely to be. Surgery on the eye muscles is undertaken as a last resort. Vision therapy may be required to get the eyes working together properly in squint cases.

Nystagmus

A defect in the visual pathway or in the eyes themselves (glaucoma, childhood cataract, and retinal problems are examples) can lead to involuntary oscillations of the eyes from side to side, up and down, or even in a circular motion. This is called nystagmus. It can begin in adulthood or childhood. Albino children and those with Down's syndrome are particularly prone to nystagmus. Adults with the condition tend to

have a constantly moving image, but the brains of the young adapt to the eye movement much better.

Nystagmus is associated with poor vision, and some affected children may be partially sighted or blind. Even those with relatively good vision might have problems with some tasks, such as reading; they may tire easily and may need a magnifier.

CHILDREN AND SCHOOL

Children with major visual problems can learn very well whether they are in mainstream or special schools. The key is to identify the visual need and then to provide appropriate resources and teacher support.

On the other hand, children with minor undiagnosed visual problems, often not picked up in a school sight test, can have specific learning difficulties that are not appreciated as being sight-related. Distance vision, peripheral awareness, and hand-eye coordination are all important in sports, for example, and near vision and eye movement skills are essential for reading. Common signs of vision-related learning difficulty include

• complaints that words are blurring;
• wobbling of the words;
• frequently losing the place on the page when reading and needing a line marker;
• problems remembering what has been read; and
• fatigue or headache when doing close work.

Some children with sight problems may be dyslexic, but sight problems are by no means the main cause of

Top of the form
Identifying and correcting any vision problems can make all the difference between being able to participate fully in classroom activity and not—crucial when it comes to happy and productive school days.

45

dyslexia. Sight-related learning difficulty and dyslexia are two different things that overlap. For example, the reading ability of children with Irlen syndrome (scotopic sensitivity) is vastly improved by the use of tinted glasses or colored overlays on the printed page. The glare on the page and the blurring and jumbling of the letters clear up with this simple device.

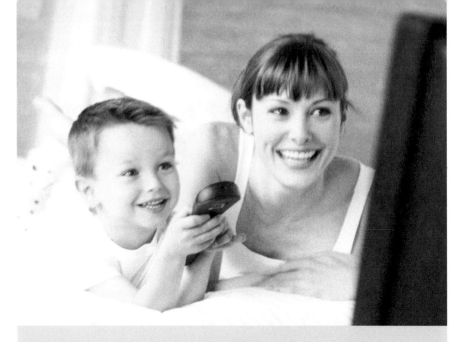

CHANGES IN ADULT VISION

Eyesight in early adulthood generally remains stable, but as people grow older it is normal for their eyesight to begin to deteriorate.

Presbyopia

Young children can sit with their noses pressed to the TV and still they see a clear image; those over 40, however, find it more and more difficult to do close work, and even reading can become difficult. This is called presbyopia, and it is only a matter of when, not if, it occurs. The lens enlarges throughout life and hardens as it does so. Presbyopia is accompanied by loss of the accommodative ability to distort the lens and focus on near objects. When it happens, you need to get reading glasses from a qualified optometrist. Glasses optimize the sight you have—they do not affect presbyopia, and lens hardening may progress, so it is important to get routine optometry checkups every couple of years.

When you need better lighting

Good lighting becomes increasingly important both at home and in the workplace as we become older. This need for better lighting has to do with pupil sluggishness and poor

WARNING SIGNS OF VISION PROBLEMS

A parent who notices any of the following symptoms in a child should schedule an eye examination: There is probably no problem, but it is better to be sure.

- Holding books close to the eye or sitting too close to the television.
- Underachieving at school.
- Blinking excessively.
- Unwillingness to read.
- Squinting or screwing up the eyes to see.
- Headaches.
- Knocking things over or bumping into things and general clumsiness.

transmission of light through the lens. As the eye ages, the pupil reacts more slowly and inadequately to changes in light. Consequently, older people tend to be more easily dazzled when exposed to bright light and take a longer time to adjust to being in the dark; this increases the risk of an accident.

How pregnancy affects the eyes

Pregnancy can have an effect on the refraction of the cornea, making vision poorer. Usually, this effect is lost soon after the baby's birth, and sight returns to normal. But any blurring accompanied by headaches and sensitivity to light should be reported to the doctor, because these can be symptoms of pregnancy-associated hypertension.

Dry eyes (see page 138) occur when there is not enough tear fluid on the eye's surface. Some women suffer from severe dry eyes when pregnant, which may make wearing contact lenses difficult.

Puffy eyelids, related to water retention, can be an uncomfortable side effect of pregnancy; cutting out caffeine and eating less salt may help reduce the severity of the swelling.

COMMON PROBLEMS AMONG OLDER ADULTS

As time passes, the risk of developing glaucoma, cataracts, or age-related macular degeneration (AMD) increases—these eye problems are all common among older people. In addition, diabetic retinopathy can be a problem for diabetics (see page 138). Cataract is the main cause of blindness worldwide, whereas AMD dominates the causes of blindness in people over age 50 in the West. Most people, if they live

There is a threefold reduction in the light reaching the retina of a 60-year-old compared to that of a 20-year-old.

long enough, will develop an age-related eye condition. Almost 30 percent of Americans over 75 are at risk for AMD, and more than half of all cataracts develop by age 50. People over 45 are at higher risk for glaucoma.

Glaucoma

Almost 60 million Americans are at risk for glaucoma, and up to half of the people with glaucoma do not know they have the disease.

The form of glaucoma most common in the U.S. is open-angle glaucoma (see page 139). This is treatable in that the eye pressure–induced loss of visual field (tunnel vision) associated with the condition can be halted or slowed down by the use of eye pressure–lowering medications. Eye drops need to be used daily for life; if drops fail, surgery is an option with a high success rate. If glaucoma is identified early, the outlook is good, but if it is recognized late, the outcome is more problematic. There is currently no way of reversing the visual field loss; treatment is directed toward saving remaining sight.

Cataract

Early in life, changes take place in the center of the lens, making it opaque. Initially, the opaque area is small and of no real consequence, but with passing years, the opacity spreads. By 65 years of age, many people have some degree of cataract. No medication has yet been found to reverse or halt the progress of a cataract, but the opaque lens can be removed surgically, if necessary, to restore vision. Using keyhole surgery techniques, the introduction of a plastic lens into the eye does away with the need for unsightly cataract glasses that were once common.

Age-related macular degeneration

AMD (see page 134) involves either a rapid or, more common, a slow developing loss of central vision because of a failure of the macula on the retina to function properly. Eventually, the macula withers and dies, so the end result is no central vision at all.

It appears that AMD is very much on the increase in the West, and it is by far the main cause of blindness or partial sight. As yet, there is no treatment for the vast majority of sufferers, although there is intense research and development underway. Although it remains a poorly understood condition, it is clear that AMD does not affect all groups of people to the same extent: It is rare, for example, in Africa and the Far East. Lifestyle and diet are factors: It is thought that exposure to excessive bright light (looking at the sun or at the light from a photocopier, for example) and smoking bring on AMD, whereas some studies have shown that dietary antioxidant vitamins (A, C, and E) delay its onset. For quality of life, it is important that AMD sufferers make best use of what sight is left, and that means getting appropriate support and advice, having good lighting, and using visual aids.

Other disorders

Dry eyes are a concern of many older people. Using an artificial tear preparation when the eyes feel particularly gritty can help.

Problems with eyelids also become increasingly likely with advancing age. Drooping of the upper eyelid (ptosis) can occur because of loss of both elastic and fatty tissue. In extreme cases, when vision is affected, surgery is the answer.

Surgery is also the solution when eyelashes on the lower lid turn inward, irritating and damaging the cornea (entropion, see page 138), or turn outward, leading to teary eyes and a greater chance of eye infection.

Are floaters harmful?

Sometimes, especially when people are tired or look at bright objects, they see small dark shapes floating across their visual field. These "floaters" are small lumps of vitreal collagen that gather when the aging vitreous starts to split away from the retina and liquefy. Floaters are more prevalent at an earlier age in people who are nearsighted or who have eyes that are larger than normal. Floaters are innocuous unless there is a sudden abundance of them: This is a sign that a retinal detachment may have taken place, and it should be treated as an emergency.

ASK THE EXPERT

Coping with failing sight

Failing eyesight can be a distressing and depressing condition, often made worse by fear or ignorance. But there is a lot of help, and an enormous number of resources are available to maximize useful vision.

GETTING HELP

When sight starts to fail, it is important to know that there is an enormous amount of help available to ensure that an individual continues to live as independently as possible.

A visit to an optometrist (optician) is a first step. An optometrist may be able to determine the cause of any change or may refer a patient to his or her physician, who can make a referral to an ophthalmologist. Sometimes the cause of vision loss is reversible. For example, a cataract can be removed and the lens replaced. The most common cause of vision loss in older people, however, is age-related macular degeneration (AMD, see page 134). A patient will be referred to an ophthalmologist if treatment is required or if vision has deteriorated to the extent that an individual can be classified as "partially sighted" or "blind."

Government assistance

Unlike countries such as England, which has a national health service, the United States does not have a national registry for the blind. Those classified as "legally blind" in the United States must rely on the state in which they live to provide certain services. Most states offer separate services for older citizens and for children.

In general, to qualify for benefits and services from the government, you must contact your state's Bureau of Disability Determination or its variation thereof. Officials at the bureau will determine, with the assistance of your doctor and other necessary medical personnel, whether your disability is severe enough to merit aid from the government. Legal blindness is defined as when the best corrected visual acuity is 20/200 or the person's visual field is 20 degrees or less. However, in some states, a person may be considered blind when his or her vision problems prevent certain activities, such as driving.

Most states focus aid on making the individual as independent as possible, which includes monetary assistance, in the form of Social Security, or rehabilitation services. Some have special programs to help visually impaired persons find employment; employers who hire through these services are often given tax credits. They sell or offer

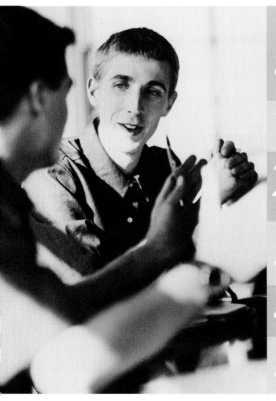

5 Ways to lend a helping hand

Because so much of our day-to-day communication involves visual cues and facial expressions, people are often unsure how to act toward a person who is visually impaired. The points below will help the sighted interact better with someone with a sight problem.

1 When talking to someone who is visually impaired, speak in a normal tone and address him or her directly—he or she is neither stupid nor deaf. Look at him or her as you would a sighted person; this makes your voice more audible and also helps the person locate you.

2 When walking, allow the person to take your arm—say whether it is your left or right—so that he or she can respond to your motion. Never take someone by the elbow and attempt to "steer" him or her. Walk at a normal pace but hesitate before stepping up or down steps or curbs. When leaving, ensure that he or she is facing the direction he or she wants to go.

3 When giving directions, don't point—it's a natural reaction, but it doesn't help. Describe the location of buildings in relation to the direction the person is (or will be) facing—for example, to your left, or at 3 o'clock. Use the number of blocks the person must walk or the number of street crossings, and use street names.

4 When showing someone to a chair, place his or her hand on the back of the chair and allow him or her to sit without guidance unless requested. His or her touch will allow him to judge the type and height of the chair.

5 In general, don't assume that the person will be unable to carry out a task. Always ask if help is required before providing it. Many vision-impaired people are highly independent.

adaptive devices to blind persons and provide vision assessment, sometimes in the person's home.

Many urban libraries offer services throughout the state to the visually impaired in the form of talking, braille, and large-print books and have a special division catering to the needs of the physically disabled. All services, including mailing for homebound patrons, are free. The Library of Congress runs the National Library Service for the Blind and Physically Handicapped (NLS), which also provides free services.

Contact your state's social services or employment office for more information.

OTHER SERVICES

An enormous range of benefits exists, although seeking out services and information can be daunting.

Low-vision aid assessment

Detection is the first step in getting help for any health problem, so many states, such as Idaho and Pennsylvania, offer vision assessment clinics. If necessary, the clinic personnel will visit your home for the appointment, which is free. The aim of the doctor is to assess what assistance the person needs in the form of adaptive devices such as lighting and magnifiers.

MAKING CHANGES

Generally speaking, there are three ways in which remaining sight can be used more effectively:
- increasing image size (or the visual field or peripheral vision),
- improving lighting, and
- increasing contrast.

Making objects appear bigger

Increasing the size of the image (that is, the image of the object on the retina inside your eye) can be achieved in three ways:
- Low-vision aids can magnify the image optically or electronically.
- Moving closer to the object will make it easier to see.
- Making the object physically larger will also increase image size.

The final method is useful for objects such as dials (on the oven, for example) and buttons (on the telephone). Numbers on thermostats can be written in large letters in a contrasting colored pen, and adaptive devices that have specifically large readouts or dials for the vision impaired can be purchased.

Improving illumination

Around the home, adapting lighting for specific visual needs can make a significant difference to daily tasks and overall mobility. Good light levels are important in most locations, particularly for elderly people. Also crucial, however, is the location of the light sources in relation to the objects being observed.

For general room lighting, it is initially important to keep light levels as even as possible, both within and between rooms. This helps minimize difficulties adapting to different light levels and coping with glare and shadows. Objects should not be placed right next to a window, because the contrast in light levels between the window and walls can cause difficulties. Overall light levels do not have to be particularly high, as long as good task lighting is available for reading and close work.

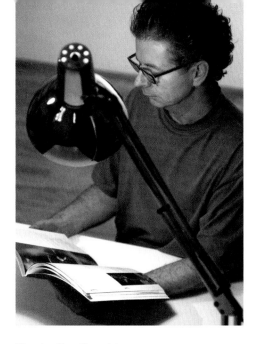

Illuminating thoughts
Reading in good daylight or by a lamp that replicates daylight can enable people with severe problems to continue to read.

Increasing contrast

Many vision-impaired people experience difficulties in detecting the outline of objects, such as the edges of tables or furniture or in locating where walls meet the floor. This obviously can affect safety as well as function and mobility. In the same way, objects are more likely to be visible and distinguishable if they differ in color or brightness from similarly shaped objects or from the surface or background on which they are located. Objects and edges can be made more visible by marking them in a contrasting color. For example, the edges of tables and light switches can be marked with bright or fluorescent tape, and flooring or walls can be light-colored to contrast with dark-colored cupboard doors. Containers for items such as sugar and milk, for example, could be selected from nonmatching sets so differences in color and shape can

Helping yourself

Making the most of remaining vision demands a combination of using every available resource and adopting vision-conscious strategies and lighting around the home. With practical advice, machinery, and gadgets, most people can adapt well to the loss of some vision.

1 Using a stick
A white stick sweeps the ground for potential obstacles and lets others know that there's a problem. Telescopic canes are easy to carry when not in use. A white walking stick helps those with mobility as well as sight difficulties; a red and white stick lets others know that there is also a hearing problem, which is vital when using the roads.

2 Harnessing touch
In the Grade 1 English version of braille, there are 63 symbols, which substitute for letters of the alphabet, punctuation marks, and numbers. Each symbol is produced by a combination of up to six raised dots arranged in two columns of three. It is estimated that less than 10 percent of the blind population is active braille users, and most of those have been blind since birth.

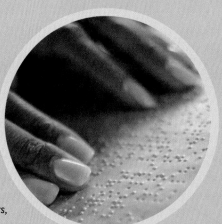

5 Fun and games
Many board and other games are available either in braille versions or with other tactile or visual cues. Playing cards, dominoes, backgammon, Scrabble, chess, and checkers are just a few familiar pastimes that can be enjoyed by all.

3 Be lens wise
Part of any low-vision assessment will involve trial and error with a range of magnifying lenses. A simple hand-held magnifier may be an appropriate aid for reading labels, but a word by word or letter by letter moving lens may be more useful for reading books and newspapers.

4 Using contrast
Dark foods on a light plate on a dark tablecloth help locate foods when eating. Placing a glass in a colored holder—or using a colored glass—makes it easier to identify its dimensions and edges. A dark cutting board is useful for locating light-colored foods and vice versa.

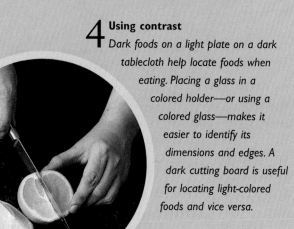

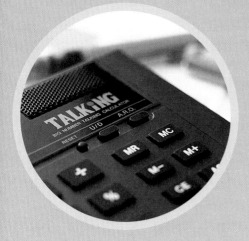

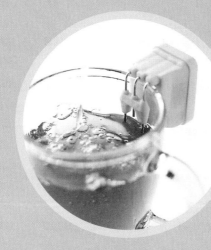

9 Beep beep
Seeing clear liquids can be tricky. Gadgets that "beep" when the liquid level reaches them can avoid potential accidents. Lots of kitchen equipment comes in visually friendly options: measuring jugs with a tactile gauge and large print or beeping timers. Raised or textured stickers can be placed on electric switches and audio controls and can be used to distinguish different settings on the oven.

10 Let's talk
Several useful gadgets are available in talking versions, including watches and clocks, calculators, kitchen scales and thermometers, and cooking timers. Many of these items are also available in tactile versions and some in braille.

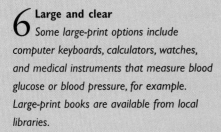

A braille book can be up to 150 times thicker than the same book in printed English.

6 Large and clear
Some large-print options include computer keyboards, calculators, watches, and medical instruments that measure blood glucose or blood pressure, for example. Large-print books are available from local libraries.

8 Braille information
For those who know braille or are motivated to learn, there is a wealth of material available. Around the house, braille label machines enable cupboard materials to be easily identified. Organizations are increasingly urged to incorporate braille on directional signs, and bank ATM machines feature braille on key pads. Some wine producers even include braille on labels.

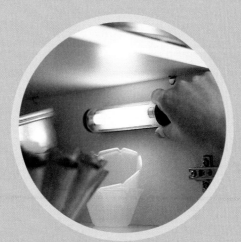

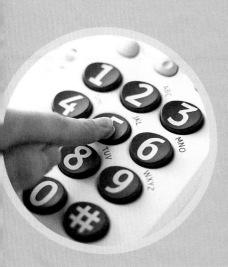

7 Lighting the way
Improving lighting is a key to maintaining the ability to read, as well as many other tasks. Task or "local" lighting should be focused as close as is practical onto the object being viewed. Ideally, a lamp should be situated in front of the plane of the person's face in order to shield the eyes from the light source and eliminate glare. Hand-held, clip-on, and flexible lights can all prove invaluable. Lights fitted inside cupboards aid product recognition.

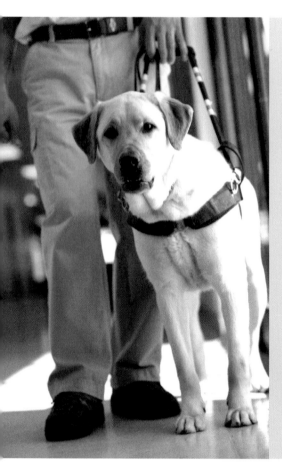

HAVING A GUIDE DOG
There are a few guide dog organizations in the United States, all of which are nonprofit. Guide Dogs of America is one of the largest. To be eligible to receive a free guide dog, a person must be over 16 and legally blind and have had previous orientation and mobility training. About 80 percent of applicants are accepted into the 4-week class. Guide dogs can usually work for 6 to 8 years, although some can work for 10, after which they are adopted.

make them more easily distinguishable. The handles of kitchen utensils or gardening tools can be marked with colored tape.

Different types of food can be placed in different-colored freezer bags (red for meat and green for vegetables) and utensils can be marked with different colored handles (a green handle for vegetable knife, yellow for potato peeler).

Large-character computer programs are available in different color combinations so that individuals can choose the background and text colors that offer the greatest contrast.

USING OTHER SENSES
The most effective intervention for the vision impaired is the optimum use of residual vision. An alternative approach is "sensory substitution," in which nonvisual senses (hearing and touch) provide an individual with information about the environment. Depending on the situation, this is used to a greater or lesser extent in conjunction with visual strategies.

Communicating
One of the most common uses for sensory substitution is for communication. "Talking books" are available from a number of sources: Many state libraries have talking book divisions, and the National Library Service for the Blind and Physically Handicapped administers a free library program of braille and audio materials to eligible borrowers in the United States via postage-free mail.

Talking books are useful for leisure but less helpful in accessing technical literature or textbooks and do not allow people to read their own correspondence. To do this, an optical character recognition (OCR) system is required. This is essentially a reading machine that can convert printed text into synthesized speech or save it on a computer.

Braille and Moon
Probably the best-known sensory substitution communication method is the braille alphabet. Although older patients can learn braille, they often find it more difficult to develop sufficient sensitivity in their fingertips. In the less-common Moon system, the embossed shapes resemble English letters.

Both Moon and braille can be written on specialized typewriters, and Moon can also be written with a penlike stylus. Books are published in both formats.

Identifying and recognizing objects
Around the home and office, the senses of touch and hearing can be used to recognize objects or gain information. Watches can be obtained that have tactile faces and hands or a vibrating mechanism that produces a series of short and long pulses for the hours and minutes. "Talking" appliances such as clocks, watches, and scales are also available. Leisure activities can be enhanced by tactile or auditory adaptations. There are balls, for example, that contain a bell to help locate them when playing sports.

Eye exercises

Eye exercises may be recommended in individual cases, such as after a stroke or a facial injury. Most ophthalmologists, however, do not subscribe to the view that the eye muscles, like other muscles, can be made to work harder.

THE BATES METHOD

Probably the best-known proponent of eye exercises as a treatment for vision problems was Dr. William Bates. After years as an eye practitioner, he observed that some of his patients noted improvement in vision without conventional treatment. His approach to eye problems was summarized in his 1920 book *Perfect Sight Without Glasses*.

Bates believed that the ability of the eye to focus did not depend on the length of the eyeball (the conventional view) but on the way the surrounding eye muscles function. Stress affects these muscles, causing vision problems. The cornerstone of Bates's philosophy is relaxation: He believed that if a person with a vision problem could relax the eye muscles and relearn how to see naturally—without tension or strain—corrective lenses would be unnecessary.

There are two components to reeducating the eye: active learning, such as when acquiring a new skill (for example, learning to paint), and receptiveness to the world. One suggested exercise is to have a "color" day, on which the patient follows a color in the environment, picking out and noting when it occurs.

Are there drawbacks?

No controlled trials have been carried out on the effectiveness of the Bates method, although there is anecdotal evidence that it works (that is, patients believe there has been an improvement in vision). However, the recommendation that a patient gets understrength corrective lenses has safety implications, as does the "sunning" technique in which patients cover their eyes and then sit or lie in the sun to relax. Accidentally opening their eyes and staring at the sun could be highly damaging. On the other hand, combatting stress through relaxation and breathing is beneficial to overall health, and in that respect, the exercises can do no harm.

Perhaps the major drawback of the method is that it can prevent people with manageable sight problems from seeking help when they should. Childhood squint, for example, can be treated but it requires intervention before a child is about 7 years old. Postponing surgery could lead to a lasting visual problem. Also, anyone with macular degeneration, cataracts, or glaucoma should seek conventional treatment.

There are training courses approved by the Bates Association, which keeps a register of those who have qualified. A teacher works one-on-one and initially is likely to recommend 6 to 10 1-hour sessions, with exercises to practice daily.

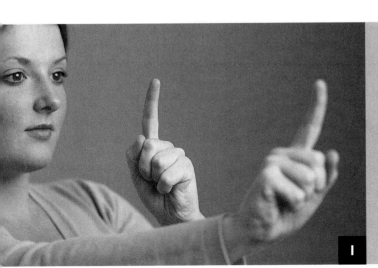

Bates's exercises

1 The technique of tromboning is advocated in the treatment of squint and astigmatism: The patient moves an object, such as a pencil or finger, backward and forward keeping it in focus at all times.

2 Palming is a key exercise intended to rest the optic nerve. With the head, neck, and eyes relaxed, a patient covers the eyes with the palms while visualizing blackness. Some teachers advocate 10 minutes a day as an adequate palming session; others believe an hour or longer to be more beneficial.

The mouth and aging

No matter what your age, you need to take good care of your teeth and mouth. Teeth and gums that are well cared for can last a lifetime and help you not only avoid a range of oral problems but also smile with confidence.

BABIES

A baby's first tooth usually appears between the ages of 5 and 7 months, although this can vary. Often, the two middle bottom teeth come through first. The process of teeth growing and breaking through the gums is called teething. Symptoms include

• fingers or fists always in the mouth;
• a swollen or puffy area on the gum;
• drooling more than usual; and
• increased crying or irritability.

To ease discomfort, babies can be given hard rubber toys or cold teething rings to chew on; teething gel may also help.

A baby's teeth should be cleaned as soon as they appear, using either a very small, soft, single-tufted toothbrush or simply a piece of damp gauze applied using a finger, and a tiny amount of low-fluoride baby formula toothpaste.

PRESCHOOL CHILDREN

Whenever possible, children should be taken to the dentist at the earliest opportunity, usually after the age of 2. Initially, a child may visit the dentist's office when a parent needs treatment, so that he or she becomes used to the environment, the dentist, and the idea that taking care of teeth and gums is important. It should be fun, so it could include a ride in the dental chair! Children can be introduced to dental care with simple procedures such as teeth cleaning. A parent or guardian should be present to consent to treatment for any minor.

Teaching children how to brush their teeth

Because children don't develop the fine motor skills needed to use a toothbrush properly until around the age of 7, they should be supervised while brushing. One way to do this is to stand behind the child and hold the toothbrush hand as he or she brushes, or you could do a "top-off" brush once the child has finished. Children should be encouraged to brush twice a day, once in the morning and once at night, using a pea-sized amount of children's toothpaste.

SCHOOLCHILDREN

Increased activity during the "growing up" years increases the likelihood of tooth damage caused by falls or being hit in the mouth.

If a tooth gets knocked out, pick it up by the crown (the part that's seen in the mouth). If the tooth is clean, place it back into its socket (the hole). If the tooth is dirty, wash it briefly in water or milk and place it back in its socket. If you can't replace the tooth, place it in a glass of milk. Get the child to a dentist immediately with the tooth; the best results are obtained when a dentist is seen within half an hour. If the tooth is chipped or broken, find the tooth fragment, place it in water or milk, and go to the dentist immediately— it may be possible to "glue" the tooth back together.

0–10 YEARS

Children lose their first teeth anyway, so why is it important to take care of them?

Children should be educated to take care of their teeth from a very early age. It is far easier to maintain good oral health-care habits learned in childhood than to try to change bad habits when the permanent teeth begin to come through. If young children need to have decayed first teeth extracted, the teeth on either side of the gap tend to drift and close up the space. This can cause a problem, because there may not be enough room for the permanent teeth to come through. In some cases, a permanent tooth may be absent or it may be developing in such a position that it is very unlikely to ever erupt in the mouth. In these instances, the adjacent primary tooth may be retained in the mouth for many years, often well into adulthood—but only if it is in good condition.

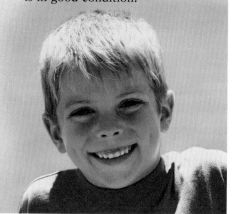

TEENAGERS

Many teenagers have orthodontic treatment to straighten crowded or irregular teeth or to correct jaw problems. Early treatment can save the need for later treatment or make the outcome of later treatment more successful. If orthodontic treatment is being carried out, it's important to
• keep the teeth very clean;
• avoid damage in sports activities;
• look out for swollen gums; and
• limit intake of acidic food or drink.

Mouth guards

Anyone who plays contact sports or a sport in which the mouth may be hit should wear a mouth guard. This applies to training sessions as well as matches. Although ready-made mouth guards can be bought from pharmacies and sports stores, a fitted mouth guard from the dentist offers the best protection. Mouth guards are available in many different colors, including purple and black!

Wisdom teeth

Wisdom teeth tend to come through between the ages of 17 and 25. Problems arise when there is not enough room in the mouth for the teeth to grow into a normal position. While they grow, a teething gel can relieve pain. A mouth rinse may also help keep the area free of bacteria and infection. For many, however, the solution is to remove the wisdom teeth.

ADULTS

Neglect rather than age causes teeth to deteriorate. It is important to have a routine of daily cleaning and regular visits to the dentist to keep your oral health. Toothaches are the most common cause of facial pain,

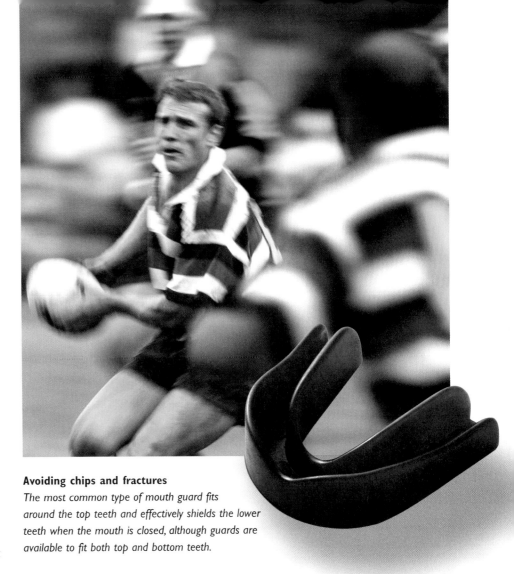

Avoiding chips and fractures
The most common type of mouth guard fits around the top teeth and effectively shields the lower teeth when the mouth is closed, although guards are available to fit both top and bottom teeth.

and most adults show signs of gum disease. Gum disease affects about 80 percent of adults. Lifestyle factors such as drinking (page 74), smoking (page 75), and stress (page 77) can also seriously affect the condition of the teeth.

OLDER PERSONS

Doctors used to think that dry mouth was a normal part of aging. This has now been disproven—older, healthy adults should not have a problem with saliva. However, older people are often prescribed medication that can cause dry mouth as a side effect. A doctor may be able to change medication or dosage if this is a problem. A dry mouth can increase the risk of tooth decay and candidiasis (oral thrush) and lead to altered taste

perception. In addition to this, the number of taste buds decrease with age and those that remain are less efficient at differentiating tastes. If food starts to taste bland, people can easily lose interest in food and end up with a diet lacking an adequate balance of nutrients.

With age, the gums may recede and teeth may become a little more sensitive as a result. The roots of the teeth can become exposed, leading to rapid erosion of the dentin. Periodontal disease may lead to the loss of teeth.

Mouth ulcers are more common in older people because of broken teeth, poorly fitting dentures, or sharp pieces of food. If an ulcer does not heal within 2 to 3 weeks, see a dentist.

Personal oral hygiene

The best way to reduce the risk of common dental diseases is to pursue a high standard of personal oral hygiene and to understand the processes that cause plaque and tartar buildup, tooth decay, and gum disease.

TOOTH BRUSHING

Tooth brushing is the principal way most of us maintain dental health. Generally, people who brush their teeth more often will have less severe gum disease than those who brush less frequently. The link between tooth brushing and tooth decay is not entirely straightforward, however; a number of other factors, such as diet and exposure to fluoride, are also involved. The quality of brushing is also crucial. Most people brush their teeth simply to make the "mouth feel clean," but this may not be enough to ensure healthy teeth and gums.

Choosing a toothbrush

Many different types and designs of brushes exist, although all fall into one of two categories: manual and electric toothbrushes.

In the manual category, most dentists recommend a brush with a short head and multiple tufts of soft or medium-textured nylon bristles. The short head makes it easier to brush more inaccessible areas.

Most electric toothbrushes have a small round head that rotates or oscillates when switched on. Although the small head can make cleaning between the teeth easier, the vibration can take some getting used to and may put some people off.

It is important to change your toothbrush or toothbrush head before the bristles become frayed. Old toothbrushes are ineffective and can harbor harmful bacteria.

Tooth brushing—how often?

Brushing twice a day is a reasonable average, although it may be better to have one very thorough session of brushing for plaque removal—about 4 to 5 minutes every day—and then a second, less thorough session to "freshen up." The thorough cleaning can be at any time that is convenient.

How to use a toothbrush

In order to make sure you are brushing your teeth effectively, it is best to use a recommended technique. One of the best manual brushing techniques is to hold the bristles at an angle of about 45 degrees to the tooth so that they point into the gap between the tooth and the gum. Move the brush backward and forward or rotate it in a circular motion using firm but gentle pressure—do not scrub the teeth and gums. A final flick of the head of the brush away from the tooth and gum will ensure the plaque is removed from the teeth.

When using an electric brush, you only have to turn it on, apply the head to the tooth surface, and then move the head slowly around your mouth rather than making the backward and forward rotating or scrubbing movements that are used with a manual brush. Remember to be gentle—the head of the electric brush is doing the work for you.

positive health tips

Tooth brushing

You should always ask your dentist or hygienist whether your tooth brushing is effective, but the following tips might be useful in the meantime:

- Select a medium- or soft-textured brush with a small head.

- Follow a routine for brushing, starting in the same place and working around the mouth to ensure that all tooth surfaces are cleaned.

- Don't leave the inside surfaces of the lower back teeth until last. Because these are the most difficult to clean, they deserve special attention when you start brushing.

- Don't forget to brush the top surfaces of your back teeth—the molars and premolars.

- Ask your dentist or water supplier about the level of fluoride in your water and use a toothpaste containing fluoride if your dentist recommends it.

Dental hygiene products

In addition to toothbrushes and toothpastes, there are a number of dental hygiene products to help you clean between your teeth. Most of these are available from pharmacies and supermarkets, although your dentist is also likely to sell them and should be able to give you advice on which might be best for you.

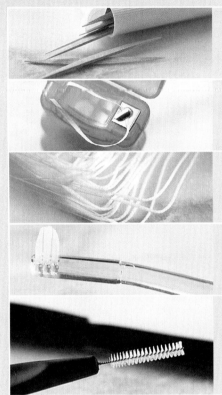

WOOD STICKS Often referred to as toothpicks, these should only be used when there is sufficient space between the teeth to accommodate them. They are much easier to use at the front of the mouth than between the back teeth.

DENTAL FLOSS Flossing demands both time and dexterity, but it is very effective for cleaning between teeth where there is not enough space for a brush or toothpick. Floss holders and threaders are available for those who find flossing difficult to master.

SUPERFLOSS This is purposely designed to clean around and beneath bridges. It has floss has a rigid part for threading and a central length of "sponge" for cleaning larger surface areas.

SINGLE-TUFTED TOOTHBRUSH Also called an interspace brush, this is a single tuft of bristles on a narrow handle and is designed for cleaning in the spaces between teeth. It is also very useful for cleaning the surfaces of teeth that show signs of gum recession.

BOTTLE BRUSH A bottle, or interdental, brush is one of the best ways to clean between teeth when there is sufficient space. These are miniature versions of the brushes used to clean test tubes and are now available in many different shapes and sizes. Again, they may be more difficult to use between the back teeth, but the brushes are available with different handles to make cleaning this part of the mouth easier.

TOOTHPASTES

Tooth brushing with toothpaste is almost certainly more effective than brushing with water alone. One function of toothpaste is to help freshen the mouth, but there are a number of other important reasons why you should use a toothpaste.

- Most toothpastes contain "active" agents that kill the bacteria in plaque or help prevent the plaque from mineralizing into tartar.
- Some toothpastes contain agents that help desensitize teeth that may become painful on contact with hot and cold drinks and cold air and when teeth are brushed—for so-called "sensitive" teeth.

- The vast majority of toothpastes now contain fluoride, which helps reduce tooth decay.
- Toothpastes help remove stains from the teeth.

What's in a toothpaste?

The main constituents of any toothpaste are the following:

- The active or therapeutic agent. These vary by product, although the most common are strontium chloride, sodium fluoride, zinc citrate, and sodium monofluorophosphate.
- The polishing agent. This is a mild abrasive that helps remove both plaque and stain.

- A binding agent to control the consistency of the paste and allow it to be squeezed easily from the tube.
- A foaming agent that helps give the paste a froth.
- An agent to prevent moisture loss and that may also add sweetness.

"Striped" toothpastes separate some of these ingredients.

A natural alternative

Before commercial toothpastes were developed, people used a mixture of equal parts of sea salt and bicarbonate of soda to neutralize bacterial acids and stimulate the gums. Modern toothpastes are much more effective for everyday use.

DAILY TOOTH CARE REGIMEN

Good brushing habits from childhood will help preserve tooth and gum health into old age. Using dental floss ensures that all surfaces of the tooth are cleaned of plaque. Although it takes a little practice and most people find it difficult to get used to, flossing is an important part of daily tooth and gum care.

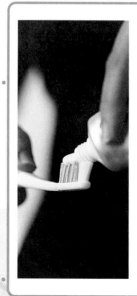

Brush teeth twice daily using a toothpaste containing fluoride and a soft- or medium-bristled brush. Hard bristles can erode the surface of the tooth and traumatize the gums, and so are best avoided.

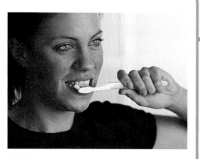

Hold the brush at a 45-degree angle to the teeth. Move the brush in short back-and-forth strokes across each tooth. Repeat this on the inside of the teeth and on the chewing surfaces.

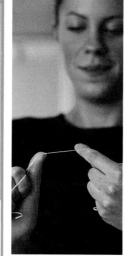

Wind the floss around your two middle fingers and pivot the central part of the floss on the thumb of one hand and the forefinger of the other to enable close control of the floss.

The floss should then be placed carefully between two teeth. Move the floss up and down against the surface of one tooth and then the other until both surfaces are clean.

MOUTHWASHES

A wide range of mouthwashes are available. Although some are designed to loosen plaque before brushing, most are used to help prevent plaque from building up on the teeth in the first place.

All mouthwashes contain an active agent, and those that contain chlorhexidine are by far the most effective in reducing, and sometimes almost eliminating, plaque formation. Mouthwashes are most useful on those occasions when it might be difficult or perhaps uncomfortable to brush the teeth—for example, when there is a viral infection or ulcers in the mouth.

Mouthwashes should only be used for relatively short periods at a time—for 1 or 2 weeks at the most. When used over longer periods, some can affect taste, and those that contain chlorhexidine will stain the teeth an unsightly brown color. Only a dentist or hygienist can remove this stain.

BREATH FRESHENERS

Although fresh breath products are fine for a "quick fix," mints and breath sprays can only camouflage bad breath for about 15 minutes. Breath products do not destroy the volatile sulfur compounds (VSCs) that cause unpleasant mouth odors. VSCs are released by bacteria that accumulate in the mouth, so the best way to freshen breath is to floss regularly and keep the teeth clean.

Chewing gum containing xylitol can inhibit bacterial growth. Studies have shown that chewing this type of gum three to five times a day for at least 5 minutes can control the growth of odor-causing bacteria.

Since 1981, the number of adults ages 55 to 64 missing all their natural teeth has declined from 33 percent to 20 percent.

BACTERIA IN THE MOUTH

The mouth is a fertile breeding ground for millions of bacteria and, no matter how well you brush your teeth, you will never create a completely germ-free oral environment. This is perfectly normal, but problems begin when the bacteria are provided with too many nutrients too often or are left undisturbed to multiply on the tooth surfaces. In these circumstances, they are much more likely to cause tooth decay and gingivitis.

What causes a coated tongue?

Tiny food particles, dead cells, and bacterial buildup get caught in the crevices of the tongue and coat it, usually with a whitish fur. A dry mouth, smoking, and mouthwashes that contain alcohol can all make matters worse.

The tongue can be gently brushed with a toothbrush to remove or reduce the coating. It is also possible to buy tongue scrapers, but when using these, it is important not to drag hard across the tongue—this could damage the taste buds.

It is normal to have a coated tongue occasionally. If it lasts for months and brushing doesn't help, see your dentist or doctor.

What is dental plaque?

Dental plaque forms continuously on teeth. It is mainly made up of bacteria that break down sugars in the diet to form a substance called a matrix, which sugars use to bind themselves both to each other and to the teeth. When plaque builds up over 1 or 2 days, the bacteria present belong to those species that cause dental caries. If the plaque is left undisturbed for longer periods of time, other bacteria, which are key in causing gingivitis and gum disease, will predominate.

Dental plaque forms not only on teeth but also on fillings, crowns, bridges, and even dentures. Thick layers of plaque can be seen as a white or yellow film with the naked eye, although thinner deposits can be seen more easily using plaque-disclosing tablets. Plaque can always be removed using a toothbrush, but this can be a difficult task when the deposit has formed in inaccessible sites such as between the teeth and just below the gum line.

What is dental calculus?

When dental plaque is left undisturbed for days (or sometimes weeks) it will start to mineralize, using the calcium and phosphate ions that are present in saliva. At first, small crystals begin to form, and these grow to form a large mass of calculus, which is also called tartar. The crystals lock tightly into very small irregularities on the tooth surface, which means that calculus cannot be removed simply by brushing; it must be removed professionally by scaling. The rate of formation of calculus can vary greatly, so some people need scaling treatment more often than others.

Calculus itself does not actually cause dental caries or gum disease, but plaque forms beneath ledges of calculus and can be difficult to remove. Calculus also has a thin film of bacteria and plaque on its surface. It is not, therefore, conducive to oral health.

IT'S NOT TRUE!

"White teeth means healthy teeth"

The natural color of the teeth is determined largely by the relative thickness of the enamel and dentin layers that make up the tooth structure. Very few natural teeth are white; their color is more often made up of a mixture of different hues and shades, and the edges of teeth can actually appear glasslike and translucent. As you grow older, the amount of dentin beneath the enamel becomes thicker, and consequently, teeth become darker, sometimes with a yellowish hue.

When dental decay begins to develop, it does so deep in the fissures on the tooth surface or between the teeth where one tooth touches another. Early dental decay is virtually impossible for you to detect by looking in your mouth and will not produce a change in color of the main tooth surface. With the passage of time, the decay becomes more extensive and the affected surface of the tooth can actually become whiter and "chalky" in appearance.

Bacteria and dental caries

Bacteria such as streptococci and lactobacilli are key in causing tooth decay, although the environment in which they exist also influences its development. These bacteria are very efficient at breaking down sugars in food; as this happens, the pH in the mouth falls, creating an acidic environment. Such acidic conditions cause the calcium and phosphate ions from tooth enamel to dissolve in a process called demineralization. This happens every time a high-sugar or high-carbohydrate meal, snack, or drink is consumed.

How do dental records help the police identify bodies?

Teeth are the hardest substance in the body, lasting even longer than bone. This means that the teeth can survive even when a body has decomposed or has been burned beyond recognition. The unique configuration of a person's teeth can help establish the identity of a body in a similar way to fingerprint or DNA evidence. Police compare the forensic information from the dental remains with the dental records of victims, including dental charts, X-rays, and plaster models of the teeth. The number of teeth, the arrangement of the teeth in the jaws, and the number and type of fillings are checked for a positive match. Unlike fingerprints, there is a record of the teeth of everyone who has ever visited a dentist.

ASK THE EXPERT

However, this is not a one-way process. While the enamel is in a highly reactive state, the calcium and phosphate ions contained in saliva actually help remineralize tooth enamel. The presence of fluoride (in tap water, for example) also aids this process and makes the tooth enamel more stable.

Fortunately, the initial mineral loss is not actually from the surface of the enamel but from a layer just below the surface. This means that, if it is diagnosed early, a dentist can apply a treatment containing fluoride to the affected surface to encourage remineralization.

Bacteria and gum disease

The bacteria in plaque are only one, albeit an important, factor in causing tooth decay, but they are of almost singular importance in causing gum problems, gingivitis and periodontal disease in particular. When plaque builds up on teeth, the environment becomes much more suited to those bacteria that thrive where there are low levels of oxygen, and these species are instrumental in causing gum problems. They start the process by releasing waste products and other chemicals that pass into the gums and damage gum tissue. These chemicals also attract defense cells from the gums' blood vessels in an attempt to prevent further infection. Occasionally, the defense cells are able to contain the infection, but in some cases, there is a very complex interaction between the bacteria and an individual's inflammatory and immune systems that eventually leads to destruction of the bone that supports the teeth. This is known as periodontitis, or periodontal disease (see page 152).

FEAR OF DENTISTS

Most people are aware that a regular schedule of dental appointments is a key factor in dental health. However, the prospect of a visit to the dentist and dental treatment can provoke anxiety in people of all ages.

A common basis for this anxiety is a previous bad experience with dental treatment, often from many years previous, usually in childhood. The thought of not knowing what is going to happen and the possibility of an uncomfortable experience are also common causes of anxiety, and some people have phobias about specific aspects of the dental environment and treatment: needles, drills, extractions, or simply having something placed in their mouth.

It is important that children do not pick up on an adult's fear of dental visits. If you know that you become anxious and can't control your fear, it might be better if someone else—a close relative or friend—accompanies your child to the dentist.

Can the fear be overcome?

A genuine fear of dental treatment is a widespread problem and can be challenging to overcome. If you are anxious about treatment, tell the dentist at the outset. A gradual approach might then be adopted, starting perhaps with advice on tooth brushing and oral health education before moving on to cleaning your teeth and then perhaps a small filling. The dentist should explain what to expect during any procedure and encourage you to give a sign for work to stop if you feel too anxious.

The dental receptionist will know to allow a little extra time for an appointment for an anxious or phobic patient. Furthermore, many dentists now offer treatment under sedation to those patients they consider to be in genuine need.

VISITING THE DENTIST

For the majority of people, regular visits to a dentist will help maintain healthy teeth and oral tissues for life.

The relatively modern concept of prevention and preventive dentistry can only be practiced effectively on those who visit their dentist for checkups on a regular basis. Frequent checkups no longer imply regular dental treatment; as many of the common dental diseases, and some of the less common ones, are entirely preventable. Regular dental visits also encourage the ongoing maintenance of good oral hygiene.

Regular checkups

Many people still only visit a dentist when they believe that something is wrong—usually the presence of severe dental pain. Pain, however, is often associated only with long-standing dental disease. For those who visit the dentist regularly, dental disease can be diagnosed early and managed before adverse symptoms develop. Conversely, the absence of pain does not imply the absence of disease. For example, tooth decay in its early stages is not painful and is often diagnosed during a routine checkup as a coincidental finding on a dental X-ray. When the decay has progressed enough to cause symptoms, a filling or even an extraction may be necessary. An early caries lesion can be managed by the application of a treatment containing fluoride rather than having to resort to drilling and filling the tooth.

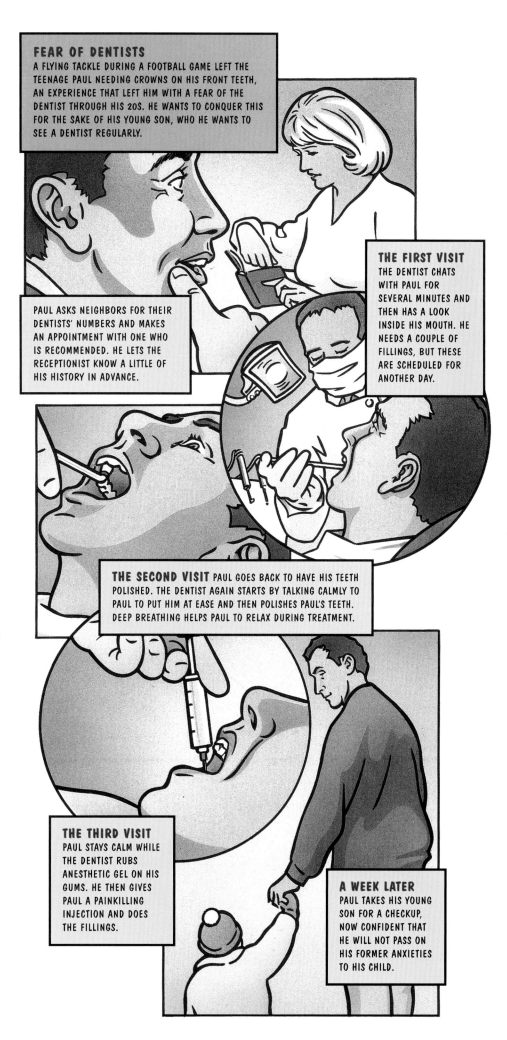

FEAR OF DENTISTS
A FLYING TACKLE DURING A FOOTBALL GAME LEFT THE TEENAGE PAUL NEEDING CROWNS ON HIS FRONT TEETH, AN EXPERIENCE THAT LEFT HIM WITH A FEAR OF THE DENTIST THROUGH HIS 20S. HE WANTS TO CONQUER THIS FOR THE SAKE OF HIS YOUNG SON, WHO HE WANTS TO SEE A DENTIST REGULARLY.

PAUL ASKS NEIGHBORS FOR THEIR DENTISTS' NUMBERS AND MAKES AN APPOINTMENT WITH ONE WHO IS RECOMMENDED. HE LETS THE RECEPTIONIST KNOW A LITTLE OF HIS HISTORY IN ADVANCE.

THE FIRST VISIT
THE DENTIST CHATS WITH PAUL FOR SEVERAL MINUTES AND THEN HAS A LOOK INSIDE HIS MOUTH. HE NEEDS A COUPLE OF FILLINGS, BUT THESE ARE SCHEDULED FOR ANOTHER DAY.

THE SECOND VISIT PAUL GOES BACK TO HAVE HIS TEETH POLISHED. THE DENTIST AGAIN STARTS BY TALKING CALMLY TO PAUL TO PUT HIM AT EASE AND THEN POLISHES PAUL'S TEETH. DEEP BREATHING HELPS PAUL TO RELAX DURING TREATMENT.

THE THIRD VISIT
PAUL STAYS CALM WHILE THE DENTIST RUBS ANESTHETIC GEL ON HIS GUMS. HE THEN GIVES PAUL A PAINKILLING INJECTION AND DOES THE FILLINGS.

A WEEK LATER
PAUL TAKES HIS YOUNG SON FOR A CHECKUP, NOW CONFIDENT THAT HE WILL NOT PASS ON HIS FORMER ANXIETIES TO HIS CHILD.

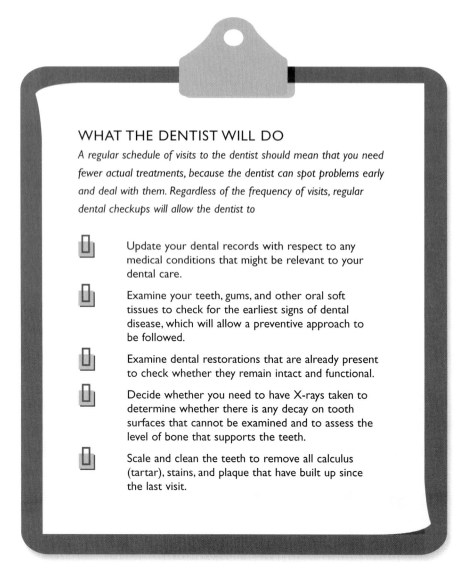

WHAT THE DENTIST WILL DO

A regular schedule of visits to the dentist should mean that you need fewer actual treatments, because the dentist can spot problems early and deal with them. Regardless of the frequency of visits, regular dental checkups will allow the dentist to

- Update your dental records with respect to any medical conditions that might be relevant to your dental care.

- Examine your teeth, gums, and other oral soft tissues to check for the earliest signs of dental disease, which will allow a preventive approach to be followed.

- Examine dental restorations that are already present to check whether they remain intact and functional.

- Decide whether you need to have X-rays taken to determine whether there is any decay on tooth surfaces that cannot be examined and to assess the level of bone that supports the teeth.

- Scale and clean the teeth to remove all calculus (tartar), stains, and plaque that have built up since the last visit.

Chronic periodontitis is caused by the bacteria that live in dental plaque, and it progresses slowly. The condition is characterized by breakdown of the ligament and bone that support the teeth in the jaws, and pain is rare. In the advanced stages of the disease, the affected teeth become loose and gaps appear between them as they move from their original positions in the jaw. To a greater or lesser extent, chronic periodontitis affects the majority of the adult population. About 10 to 15 percent of the Western adult population is affected by the advanced stages of chronic periodontitis, and many of these individuals will go to dentists for the first time, having previously been unaware of any dental problems. At this late stage of the disease, the extraction of teeth may be inevitable, although the condition can be diagnosed and managed successfully, if not prevented altogether, in those people who visit a dentist on a regular basis.

Regular dental visits also allow the early detection of other dental problems that might be developing. The dentist will probe the gums for inflammation and tooth mobility and examine your mouth for indications of possible vitamin deficiencies or cancer. Many people are now keeping their natural teeth for life, and all teeth are subject to wear either from the physical processes of eating and tooth brushing or from acidic substances that are part of the diet. The rate of tooth wear varies, but even when the rate of progression is very slow, there is a significant possibility that teeth will show wear in later life. This problem can be very challenging for a dentist to treat and is much less difficult to prevent. Regular visits will allow dentists to detect and manage tooth wear as soon as the first signs appear.

A dental schedule

Those who visit a dentist usually do so every 6 months, and most dentists will send cards or "reminders" to encourage a twice-yearly attendance pattern. Six-month checkups became generally accepted as being appropriate for most people at a time when the prevalence of tooth decay was far greater than it is today. Dental treatment on a regular basis was essential if the ravages of tooth decay were to be kept under control by the placement, and then replacement, of fillings.

Although the pattern of dental disease has changed over the last 20 to 30 years, regular visits to the dentist should still be encouraged. As the dentist-patient relationship develops, the dentist is able to assess an individual's risk of developing dental disease based on the patient's previous dental experiences. Consequently, the dentist may determine a pattern of visits appropriate to the individual. If the risk of dental disease is low, then a visit every year may be considered, but a 3-month checkup might be sensible if the risks are high.

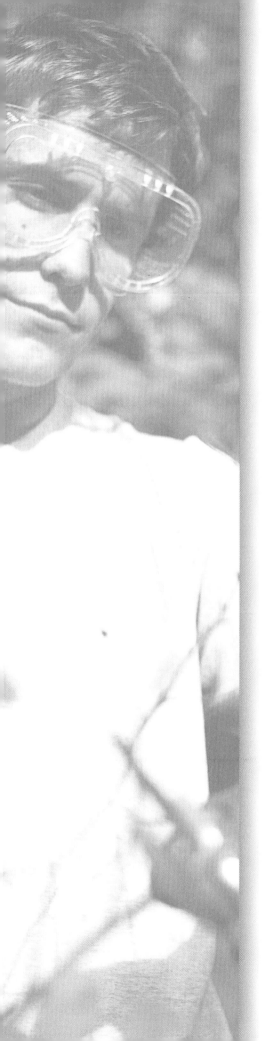

GOOD HEALTH FOR THE EYES AND MOUTH

Keeping the eyes and mouth healthy is a matter of understanding the risk factors and learning how to minimize their potential effects. This can range from simple steps such as wearing sunglasses or a mouth guard to life-changing strategies such as giving up smoking and learning to manage stress.

64 Whether at home or at work, here is how to protect your eyes from harm, plus effective first aid to minimize any accidental damage.

68 An allergic reaction can cause sore, watery eyes in susceptible individuals, but it is possible to lessen the impact.

70 The weather can have an effect on eye health. Sun and wind are particularly harmful, but light reflecting off water can also cause problems.

73 Many people are aware of the risks of alcohol on general health, but nonalcoholic drinks can severely damage teeth as well.

75 Smoking is responsible for many oral problems, from cosmetic complaints such as stained teeth to cancer of the mouth, lips, or throat.

77 Stress can cause oral problems, including dry mouth, ulcers, and cold sores, but self-help techniques can control stress and its effects.

Healthy eyes at work and home

Just as it is in the workplace, eye injury is all too common in the home and during leisure activities, particularly in connection with "do it yourself" projects, gardening, car maintenance, and sports.

Many accidents at work occur either because eye protection was inappropriate or, more often, because although protection was available, it was not used or not used correctly; an unreasonable risk was taken that should not have been taken.

In their own homes, people often tend to be unaware of the hazards around them and may not realize that they are putting themselves at risk. A do-it-yourself (DIY) enthusiast who would never be without safety goggles in the workplace may never think to use them at home or when playing sports. Ocular injury is more frequent at work than at home (70 percent of injuries occur at work as opposed to 20 percent at home), but severe eye injuries are more common in the home. In the workplace, machine tool operators record the highest number of injuries, followed by mechanics and metalworkers. Children at play and the elderly are particularly vulnerable in the home environment.

Most accidents to the eye are preventable, regardless of whether they happened at work or at home. By far, the majority of injuries are minor, but even injuries that are not sight-threatening are invariably painful and incapacitating for a while. It is worth remembering that near the surface of the cornea, there are more than 400 times as many sensory nerve endings as there are on the skin.

BLUNT INJURY

The eye socket, brow ridge, nose, and eyelids are the main external defenses that absorb much of the impact of a blow around the eye. The shape and tension of the eye also help absorb the energy of an impact. Thinking of the bruised face of a boxer after a fight may help you appreciate how effective eye defenses need to be. In some cases, blunt, or contusion, injuries are so massive that they overwhelm the natural defenses of the eye and distort the eyeball. In these circumstances, damage is caused by a wave of pressure passing through the delicate contents of the eye. Intraocular bleeding is possible, retinal detachment is a common complication, lens damage will lead to cataract, and, because of tissue displacement, glaucoma can develop. The most severe cases are associated with a fracture of the orbit, the eye socket.

In the workplace, flying projectiles, explosions, release of compressed air, a jet of fluid escaping from a burst pipe, or simply tripping and hitting a blunt object can cause contusion injuries to the eye.

At home, falls are a major cause of blunt injury but contusion damage

BEING EYEWISE
The keys to preserving eye health are to be aware of the risks and to take advantage of any safety equipment. Although the risk of blindness is generally small, painful injuries are common.

HEAT SENSE
Glass blowers traditionally risked burning injuries; eye protection is vital here and for metalworkers.

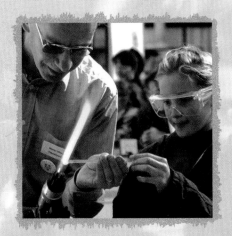

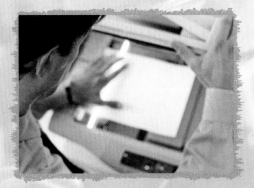

BRIGHT LIGHTS
In addition to the golden rule never to look at the sun, it is not a good idea to stare at any bright light. Never look at the light generated by a photocopier, for example, because the retina can be damaged.

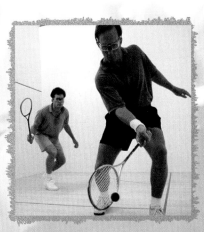

HARDBALL
A squash ball can have more force than a bullet, and both beginners and advanced players are at risk. Squash, racquetball, and paddle ball account for more than 10,000 injuries per year.

can occur from more exotic accidents. A champagne cork can cause extensive eye damage, and severe contusion injuries have been caused by inflating airbags in cars.

Players of contact sports risk contusion eye damage, and racket sports are often negatively highlighted for this type of eye injury. Squash balls have a particularly bad reputation. A ball travels at up to 140 miles per hour and in flight distorts to an oval shape that neatly fits the eye socket. A good example of what can be done to limit accidents comes from Canada. Canadian racket sports eye injuries in the 1980s were mostly caused by squash (73 percent), but this figure fell to 23 percent in the 1990s after the introduction of mandatory eye protection for squash players.

PERFORATING INJURY

Any sharp object or foreign body is a potential hazard that can impact on and even penetrate into the eye.

Foreign body injuries make up about half of all ocular traumas. Especially common objects are shards of metal, splinters of wood, and glass fragments. These materials may hit the eye and cause injury. Eye injuries from glass, however, have decreased dramatically since the introduction of seat belt legislation.

Superficial foreign bodies often become embedded under a lid, in the cornea, or in the conjunctiva and cannot be removed even by copious rinsing with water. Avoid rubbing and do not try to remove a sharp object with tweezers or such, because that can cause additional damage. Such injuries need speedy medical attention.

Perforating injuries result from sharp objects entering the eye. All cases of this type need medical care right away. Do not let the victim rub the eye and do not pad it. The eye needs to be protected and kept as clean as possible to avoid or minimize future infection, so use a

cover that protects the eye without touching it. The bottom of a lightweight plastic or cardboard cup held or taped over the eye is useful. If the eyeball is severely damaged, it may collapse and its contents—iris or vitreous—may spill out; this may cause extreme pain.

On the other hand, the sufferer may experience only nominal pain from a small projectile. Small projectiles, particularly lumps of hot metal traveling very fast, can pass into the globe and seal the entry wound on the way. There may be no external evidence at all and the object may only be picked up on clinical examination, X-ray, or ultrasound. A static, irregular pupil is a giveaway sign that there is a foreign body in the eye.

Any intraocular foreign body needs to be removed because, in addition to any damage to internal structures it may cause, there is additional risk of toxicity or infection from the material if it is left inside the eye too long. Some materials such as plastic

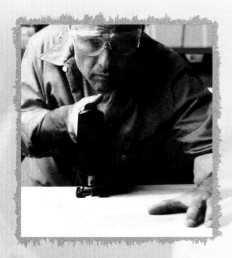

WOOD CHIP
Sanding and cutting wood or fiberboard produce dust and tiny flying chips that can cause pain. Safety goggles are a must for any DIY project involving cutting or sanding.

THINK BLINK
Computer screens are safe for the eyes, but it is vital to remember to blink and to refocus your eyes away from the screen frequently.

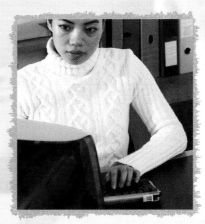

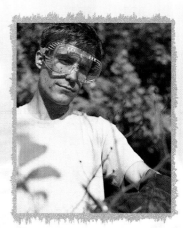

GARDEN GOGGLES
The garden presents several potential hazards for the eyes. Use eye protection when pruning—especially from below—or working around stakes and canes.

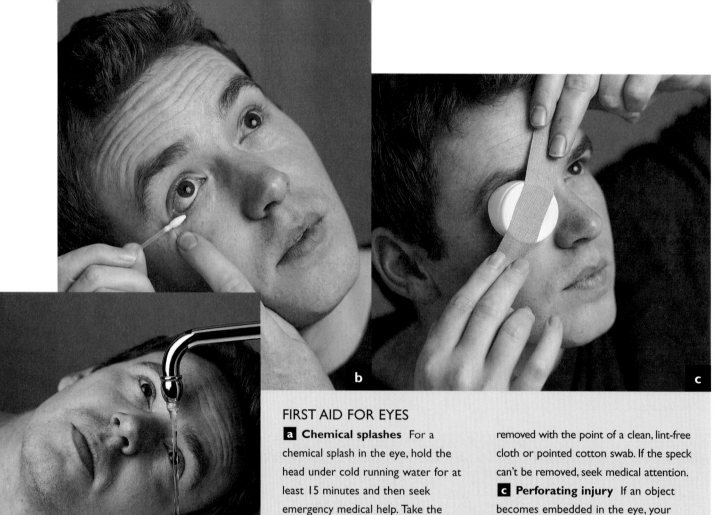

FIRST AID FOR EYES

a Chemical splashes For a chemical splash in the eye, hold the head under cold running water for at least 15 minutes and then seek emergency medical help. Take the chemical container with you if possible.

b Surface irritants Easily visible foreign objects that are clearly on the surface and not embedded can often be removed with the point of a clean, lint-free cloth or pointed cotton swab. If the speck can't be removed, seek medical attention.

c Perforating injury If an object becomes embedded in the eye, your initial goal is to prevent further damage. Cover the eye with the bottom of a paper cup, try to keep the eyeball still, and seek emergency medical attention.

and glass are well tolerated, whereas copper and iron are particularly dangerous. Copper induces severe inflammation in the eye, and when iron oxidizes, it causes a slow degeneration of the retina that leads to blindness. Wood carries with it a covering of bacteria and molds that, if carried into the eye, cause a pus-filled inflammation of the whole eye (endophthalmitis), often associated with profound visual loss. Rose thorns sometimes jab into the eye of unwary gardeners, and these injuries are always of major concern because of the high level of bacteria and molds that can find their way into the body.

A sightless eye may have to be removed if damage is severe, because there is a small risk that an immunological reaction may affect the undamaged eye—so-called sympathetic ophthalmitis. Immunosuppressive management and surgical refinements have made this condition much rarer than it once was. Several historical figures were tragically blinded by sympathetic ophthalmitis, including Louis Braille, the inventor of the writing system for the blind.

CHEMICAL INJURY

Acids and alkalis can cause corrosive burns and scarring of the eye. Of these, the injuries caused by alkalis are more extreme and are less likely to improve with time. Alkalis, such as household bleach, penetrate more easily into the eye than acids and produce profound intraocular alterations that often result in severe late complications such as corneal ulceration, neovascularization, cataract, and glaucoma. A severe chemical injury burns all the superficial blood vessels, causing a completely white and opaque eye. Corneal grafting will be required, but the success rate in such cases is poor.

Sulfuric acid from car batteries is among the more common sources of acid injuries. Sodium hydroxide (used in the chemical and pulp and paper industries) and ammonia (found in fertilizers and plastics) cause horrendous alkali burns because they penetrate into the eye very rapidly. Lime burns are all too common in the building trades.

Anyone who suffers a chemical injury to the eye must flush it immediately with copious amounts of water, preferably under a running faucet. Industrial solvents and detergents cause problems if they get into the eye. Benzene, acetone, ethanol, and tricloroethylene are common solvents in the paint, plastics, and rubber industries. Paints and thinners can also cause eye problems through DIY accidents at home.

RADIATION AND LIGHT INJURIES

Infrared is long-wavelength radiation that can penetrate throughout the eye and cause thermal injuries to the cornea, lens, and retina. Welders who do not use appropriate protection are at risk, and glass blowers in the past commonly developed a radiation cataract. Household microwave ovens carry no risk unless they are faulty.

Ultraviolet (UV) is short-wavelength radiation that does not get to the back of the eye. It can, however, produce nasty burns to the front of the eye (photokeratitis) and a photochemical-induced cataract. Gazing into an open furnace without eye protection produces photokeratitis. Injuries to arc welders are sometimes referred to as "arc eye," which causes discomfort comparable to grit or sand in the eye (see page 71).

It is known that visible light, if sufficiently intense, damages the retina, among other structures. Some ophthalmic instruments reach such levels, but exposure is short and retinal damage, if any, is easily repaired. Artificial lighting levels, are way below the acute damage threshold, but there is a theoretical risk of long-term damage. Little is known for certain on this subject, but some vision scientists are concerned that increasing light levels and our progression toward the 24-hour artificial day puts increasing demands on our eyes and offers less opportunity for repair.

LASERS

Lasers emit light of differing intensity, wavelength, and type of beam (pulsed or continuous), and in many circumstances they can be hazardous to the eyes. Lasers are classified as 1, 2, 3A, 3B, and 4, with 3B and 4 being dangerous to the eye. Industrial, military, and medical lasers are usually of the more dangerous types. Pulsed lasers, such as the Q-switched and mode-locked, are of very short duration and have an explosive pulse effect on tissues, whereas long and continuous waves will burn. Industrial laser damage to the eye ranges from minor retinal burns to extensive ocular damage and major loss of vision. Most injuries seem to be associated with failure to use appropriate safety equipment.

In recent years, there have been worries about laser pointers, widely used during presentations at conferences and other business and academic events. Generally, it is thought that because pointers are class 1, 2, or 3A lasers, they are unlikely to cause any eye injuries. However, many are being produced that are not properly classified and may be more dangerous than was thought. They are also widely available. Laser pointers, in the hands of the irresponsible, can be dazzling or distracting, and, used inappropriately, are a real hazard to drivers.

COMPUTER SCREENS

All research conducted so far suggests that computer screens do not damage eyesight but often make users aware of vision problems that they have already. Without doubt, if posture is poor, glare is high, and the operator spends long periods at the workstation, fatigue will set in. In these circumstances, it is not surprising that operators think computers are bad for their eyes.

WHAT YOU CAN DO

To protect your eyes at work and home and during leisure pursuits,

- Wear any available protective eye gear supplied by your employer correctly and in the appropriate circumstances. Make sure eye gear is tested for continued suitability and safety as recommended.
- Find out what protective eyewear is available for sports use and equip yourself. Use appropriate eye protection for DIY and gardening.
- Don't take chances. Some damage is cumulative, and a serious eye injury can happen in seconds.
- Get immediate medical help for all but the most minor injuries.
- If you suspect a vision problem, see an ophthalmologist immediately.

About 1000 eye injuries occur in workplaces every year, costing $300 million. An estimated 90 percent could be prevented by protective glasses.

Allergy and the eyes

An allergic reaction occurs when you come in contact with a substance or agent (an allergen) to which your body is sensitive. For many people, the most likely cause of allergy in the eyes is pollen, but this is just one of several causes.

THE ALLERGIC REACTION

Your body reacts to a sensitive substance by releasing histamine from defense cells—known as mast cells—in order to combat the inflammation. As a result, the affected tissue becomes red, puffy, and sore. This is particularly obvious when it involves the eyes because the skin of the lids is thin and the delicate conjunctiva is packed with reactive blood vessels.

A mild attack

For an occasional mild reaction, a cold washcloth over the eyes will reduce the discomfort. Artificial tear preparations in the form of eye drops may help until the symptoms subside.

An acute attack

The common feature of an acute ocular allergic reaction is conjunctivitis with severe swelling. The swelling, called chemosis, can be so pronounced that it extends beyond the lids and the lids themselves become puffy and red, which can be extremely uncomfortable. The eyes water and itch, and this may be accompanied by a stinging or burning sensation. This type of attack is frequently seen in children who have been exposed to too much pollen while playing in a field or too many particles from fur and skin when stroking a cat, for example. Fortunately, for most people, the response to an acute ocular allergic reaction is self-limiting and is usually over within a few hours.

When a reaction becomes chronic

For a few children and adults who are prone to hereditary asthma and eczema, an allergic eye reaction may become chronic if the sufferer is exposed repeatedly to the allergen. The condition is known as vernal keratoconjunctivitis in children and atopic keratoconjunctivitis in adults. Steroid drops should be part of the treatment if corneal ulceration is to be avoided.

Eye makeup—the cause of so many allergic reactions—was first used by the ancient Egyptians to protect their eyes from infection and sun.

COMMON TRIGGERS

A mild, seasonal allergic eye response may be triggered by pollen in the summer "hay fever" months. Eye drops with both antihistamine and blood vessel constriction actions can be used to relieve symptoms. People with a history of seasonal allergy might use sodium cromoglycate or a similar mast cell stabilizing preparation. These drops are valuable preventatives, but to be effective, they must be used every day throughout the hay fever season.

For people who suffer a non-seasonal response, the most common allergens are dust mites, fur and dry skin on pets, and bird feathers.

Other causes of ocular allergies include contact lens solutions, preservatives in eye drops, and cosmetics. In some work-related environments, such as engineering workshops and bakeries, inflammatory eye responses are common, because these jobs involve the handling of paints or textiles, for example.

In all cases, it is important that the allergen be identified and avoided, and this is not always easy. In fact, in some cases, the allergen may never be identified.

Reactions to makeup

There are ingredients in all cosmetics that can induce contact dermatitis. Because of the delicacy and sensitivity of the eye area, it is this region that most often reacts to cosmetic-derived allergens.

Makeup removers and eye creams have a reputation for inducing allergic eye inflammation. Mascara, especially the lash-building type that contains fibers that can fall into the eye, is the worst offender and best avoided if you are at all sensitive. Oil-based mascaras pose a greater risk than water-based ones, and using oily makeup removers compounds the problem.

Not just eye makeup

Rashes around the eyes and an itchy, burning sensation can occur as a reaction to beauty products other than eye makeup. For example, some perfumes can make the eyes itchy. Hair sprays and dyes, and even nail polish, have been known to cause conjunctivitis. As a precaution, you should take care to keep all aromatherapy oils away from your eyes.

Avoiding an allergy attack

The number one tip for how to avoid an allergic ocular reaction is to stay away from whatever it is that triggers the allergic response. Often, this is not possible. When this is the case, try following these tips and hints for preventing—or at least limiting—an unwanted attack.

1 Shield eyes from harm
Wear glasses or sunglasses to keep pollen out of your eyes. Some optometrists recommend not using contact lenses when pollen counts are at their highest, because the lenses can act as pollen traps.

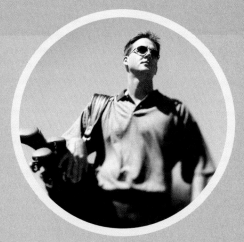

5 Wage war on dust
Where possible, replace carpets with hard-surface floors. Vacuum all floor surfaces regularly. Change your bedding frequently and vacuum the mattress from time to time.

4 Wash the family pet
Clean dogs and cats frequently to reduce the amount of dead skin (dander) they shed at other times. Many people are allergic to dander.

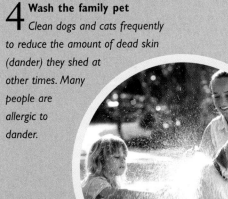

2 Wash your hands
Wash your hands frequently to avoid transferring antigens such as pollen from hand to eye when you rub your eyes. In addition, try not to rub your eyes, although this is one of those actions that we all tend to do without thinking. If you have to handle a substance to which you know you are allergic, wear protective gloves.

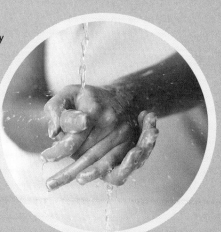

3 Makeup, lenses, and eyes
Not only are some people allergic to substances in makeup, but the act of putting on makeup can transfer other allergens to the eye area. Contact lens wearers should take particular care when handling lenses, because a lens can trap makeup that falls into the eye.

Protecting eyes from sun and wind

Our eyes are vulnerable to damage from too much sun or wind. Initially, the effect on vision may be disabling but temporary. With repeated or prolonged exposure, however, minor injuries can turn into major problems.

DANGERS FROM SUNLIGHT

We require light to see, but excessive sunlight can be extremely harmful. If you take a magnifying glass and focus the sun's rays on dry grass or paper, you will start a fire. We have the equivalent of a magnifying glass—the lens—inside our eye whose job it is to focus weak light on the retina so that we can see. Looking directly at the sun can cause retinal burns or, even more visually damaging, a burn on the macula.

Sun gazing dazzles but causes no pain, and the resultant loss of vision is delayed for several hours. Although such deliberate harm is unusual, accidents can happen while viewing an eclipse (whether partial or total). Sunglasses are not sufficient protection for staring at the sun or watching a eclipse. The only safe way to watch an eclipse is to view an indirect projection on a white card and not look directly at the sun at all.

Natural defenses

A combination of our own behavior and the location of our eyes protects them from the full glare of the sun. We avoid looking at the sun as a matter of course, and in many hot countries, people adopt a slight stoop and lowered head posture when outdoors. The eyes are also protected from sunlight injury by being placed fairly deep in their sockets and covered by the lids. This arrangement provides fairly effective sun screening. The third member of the "external defense force" is the brow ridge that shades the eye from excessive light from above.

The "internal defense force" is at least as important and serves to protect the vulnerable retina from the ravages of excessive light. The iris is of particular significance because it controls the size of the pupil and therefore the amount of light entering the back of the eye. In gloomy, conditions the pupil's diameter is a maximum of about .8 inch, whereas in the brightest light the pupil constricts to .05 inch. Iris constriction is a reflex action; when an individual is dazzled, this reaction can reduce the amount of light entering the eye 30-fold.

Pigment cells in the retina are also a crucial part of internal defense because they help protect the light-sensitive rods and cones (see page 24) by neutralizing free radicals and other light-induced chemicals that may harm the eye.

The effects of prolonged exposure

Long-term exposure to high levels of sunlight, specifically ultraviolet (UV) light, is associated with the development of several eye disorders.

- It has been suspected for some time but is not yet proven that exposure to too much light is a key factor in the development of age-related macular degeneration (AMD, see page 134).
- A pterygium is a growth of opaque tissue from the conjunctiva; this is induced by ultraviolet radiation and can grow over the cornea and distort the cornea's shape, causing vision to become impaired.
- Labrador keratopathy is a disorder in which the sun-exposed cornea and conjunctiva accumulate yellow deposits, causing loss of vision.

Blinded by the light
When sunlight is reflected by glass, water, snow, sand, roads, or any other shiny surface, the light intensity increases by as much as 20 times what it would be otherwise.

You should not stare directly at the sun, even if wearing high-quality sunglasses. The light-sensitive retinas of your eyes could still be damaged.

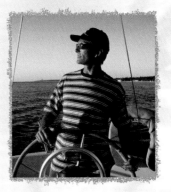

REFLECTED LIGHT FROM WATER
Special purpose sunglasses shield sailors' eyes from the glare that comes off sheets of water under hot sun.

- UV light is believed to accelerate cataract formation (see page 135).
- Long-term sun exposure can cause skin cancer, which commonly affects the eyelids; the link between sun exposure and a tumor in the eye is less clear (see page 110).

Reflected light

Humans evolved in a grassland environment where most of the risk to our eyes from sunlight came from above; reflected light levels were relatively low. In the modern city, packed with concrete and glass, reflected light levels are very high. We are protected from direct sunlight from above, but our defenses are less able to cope with reflected light from eye level and below. The effect of long-term exposure to far higher levels of reflected light than our eyes were evolved to deal with is, as yet, unknown, but many eye doctors think that it contributes to the growing numbers of elderly people with age-related macular degeneration or cataracts. Wearing polarizing sunglasses can eliminate or reduce reflected light.

Snow blindness

Acute damage caused by excessive reflected sunlight occurs in its most extreme form when the light is reflected off snow, which reflects back about 85 percent of the ultraviolet (UV) radiation within sunlight. White sand has a similar effect. This UV radiation causes the equivalent of sunburn to the cornea. Symptoms of snow blindness may not be apparent for a number of hours after light exposure. A sufferer then experiences headache and pain; very sore, sensitive eyes; and hazy vision. These symptoms persist for a couple of days and can be very alarming. The main culprit is UVB, which damages the delicate epithelium on the surface of the cornea, making the eye vulnerable to infection until the epithelial barrier reforms. A single episode is unlikely to cause long-term damage unless secondary infection sets in, but repeated or persistent exposure may permanently damage the cornea.

As protection, skiers and climbers should wear special wraparound sunglasses or goggles that prevent sunlight from getting in at the sides and have UV radiation filtering that is at least 90 percent effective.

SUNGLASSES

Sunglasses can shield your eyes from UV rays and glare, but the extent to which they do this varies. The darker the lenses, the more light is blocked out and the less glare you will see—and the darker the world will appear through the lenses—but this is not necessarily a measure of how well UV rays have been screened out.

UV radiation protection

Several organizations in many countries regulate nonprescription sunglasses. British and Australian standards are generally more strict than those in the United States.

There are two U.S. regulating agencies: the American National

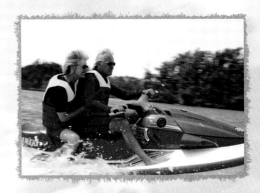

SHIELDING THE EYES FROM WIND
Wind resistance can damage the delicate surface of the eye by carrying particles into the eye at high speeds.

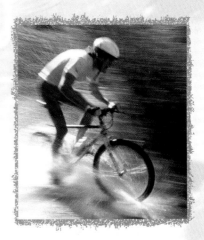

PROTECTION FROM GLARE AND SPRAY
Droplets of water can be as damaging as particles of solid matter if they hit the eye at high speed. Goggles or glasses protect from the glare reflected by sheets of water.

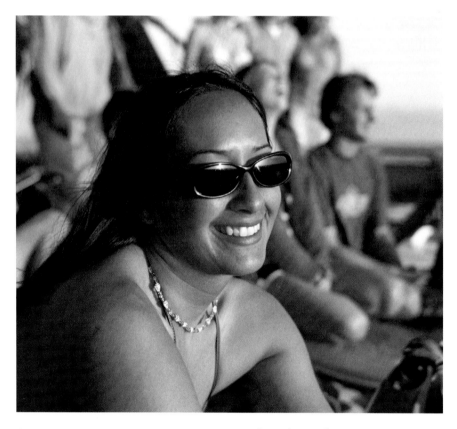

Combining good sense and glamour
Wearing sunglasses while out in the sun not only protects the retina from damage but also helps reduce premature aging of the delicate skin that surrounds the eyes.

Standards Institute (ANSI) and the Sunglass Association of America, in conjunction with the Food and Drug Administration (FDA). ANSI sets standards for cosmetic quality, refractive properties, and impact resistance. ANSI standard Z80.3–1966 divides sunglasses into three categories:

• **Cosmetic sunglasses** block at least 70 percent of UVB and up to 60 percent of UVA.
• **General purpose** sunglasses block at least 95 percent of UVB and at least 60 percent of UVA.
• **Special purpose** sunglasses block at least 99 percent of UVB and 60 percent of UVA.

If sunglasses do not meet ANSI Z80.3–1996 section 4.6.3 or International Standards Organization (ISO) Standard 14889, they must carry a caution stating, "not recommended for use while driving."

Additional choices

• **Fully tinted lenses** Lenses are one color throughout.
• **Gradient tint lenses** Each lens is darker at the top than at the bottom and thus gives protection from bright overhead light while allowing activities such as reading. Gradient lenses are not as good at protecting the eyes from dazzling sheets of water or snow, however.
• **Photochromatic lenses** These are light-sensitive lenses that darken quickly on exposure to sunlight and therefore are particularly useful when you are going in and out of doors often and don't want to be constantly taking your sunglasses off and on.
• **Polarizing lenses** These give extra protection against glare by sandwiching a special filter between two sheets of plastic or glass.

WIND DAMAGE

Often our eyes fill with tears when we are outside and in cold windy weather. These tears are produced to protect the delicate corneal surface. Some people, especially those who are older, suffer from dry eye, which means that they cannot produce sufficient tear fluid to protect their eyes. Without the natural lubrication of the tear film, the eyes become dry, reddened, itchy, and vulnerable to secondary infections. Liberal use of artificial tears (available over the counter from the pharmacist; see page 103) is advisable for people with dry eye who are spending time outside on cold windy days.

Wind and dust

Particles of dirt carried by the wind are a big problem for people who live under sandy or dusty conditions. In particular, the dry dusty winds of the desert worsen the soreness of sufferers of the eye infection trachoma (see page 145). Poor hygiene leads to a cycle of infection and reinfection that causes the cornea to become scarred and opaque. With 600 million sufferers, of whom 1 in 100 become blind, trachoma is the third most common cause of blindness in the world, after cataracts and glaucoma.

Drinking and oral health

Most of the reported links between drinking and general health are based on the intake of alcohol. The known effects of drinks on oral health, however, are associated with both alcoholic and nonalcoholic beverages.

Most alcoholic and nonalcoholic drinks contain either acid or sugar (and often both), and because of this, may be detrimental to the teeth and oral health.

WHAT IS TOOTH EROSION?

Tooth erosion is the wear of tooth surfaces caused by the action of chemicals, predominantly acids, including those that are present in drinks. There are no bacteria involved in the process of erosion, so it is a completely different condition from dental caries. Essentially, the acids soften the enamel of the tooth surface, which may be further dissolved or worn away by the action of tooth brushing (abrasion) or the teeth moving over one another during eating (attrition).

Erosion can affect the primary teeth as well as the permanent teeth, and there are many reported cases in which the teeth of young adults and even children have been worn almost completely flat. The affected teeth will become sensitive only when the tooth wear is advanced and the enamel surface has completely worn away. As the underlying dentin becomes visible, the teeth develop a darker, yellow color. When drinks are the predominant cause of the erosion, the inner surfaces (palatal and lingual) of the teeth are predominantly affected, so the loss of tooth substance may not be obvious, except to a dentist during a checkup. Erosion can also be caused by eating an excess of fresh citrus fruits: oranges, grapefruits, and in some cases, lemons. In such cases, the wear also affects the outer surfaces of the incisors and canines.

SUGARS IN DRINKS

The constituent that makes most drinks more palatable is sugar, which unfortunately also has a direct effect on the development of dental caries. The taste for sugary drinks often begins in early childhood. Fruit juices with a very high sugar content are given in bottles to infants who are allowed to pacify themselves during long periods with what is literally a continuous, sugary drip feed. Some children's medicines also have a high sugar content to make them more palatable, and many drinks that normally target young children and adolescents also contain significant amounts of sugar.

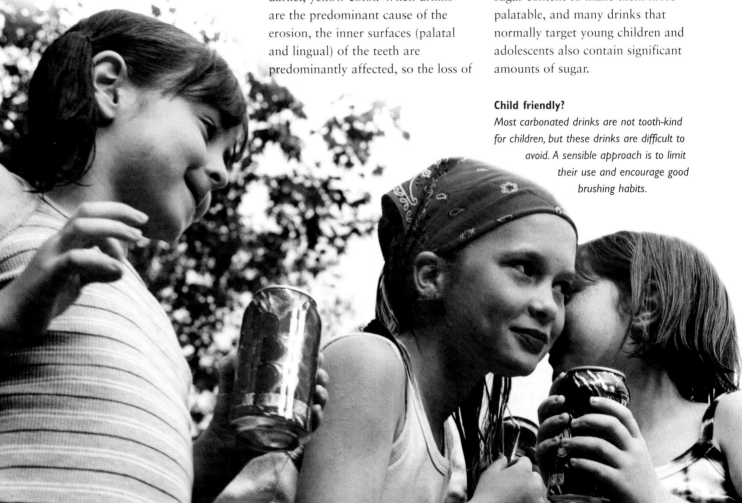

Child friendly?
Most carbonated drinks are not tooth-kind for children, but these drinks are difficult to avoid. A sensible approach is to limit their use and encourage good brushing habits.

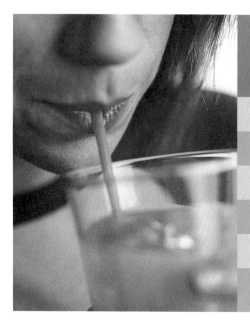

6 Hidden dangers of drinks

The principal dangers in drinks are that sugar causes tooth decay and acid causes tooth erosion. Some drinks may also stain the teeth.

1 Red wines and port have a tendency to stain the teeth; port also has a high sugar content.

2 Wines, cider, and beers contain high levels of sugar and acid. Combining alcohol with sugary or acidic snacks compounds the problem.

3 Alcohol has been proven to cause oral cancer, but it is particularly damaging in combination with smoking.

4 Carbonated or acidic drinks may cause tooth erosion. Drinking through a straw may reduce the damage.

5 Sports drinks are acidic and may also cause tooth erosion; water is the best drink for hydration during sports activities, with a sports drink at the end.

6 Diet or "light" drinks are likely to be less damaging with respect to causing caries, but some still contain measurable quantities of sugar and can still cause erosion.

STAINED TEETH

Tea, coffee, and red wines contain tannin, which will cause staining on the surface of the teeth. Heavy drinkers of these beverages will have more heavily stained teeth. The dark brown staining is harmless and can be removed by a cleaning from a dentist. Red wines and port also stain the tongue and lips. However, only the surface layer is stained and the color is quickly washed away by saliva.

THE EFFECTS OF ALCOHOL

Excess alcohol intake can result in gastric irritation and reflux, which can worsen tooth erosion. However, the most serious oral threat from drinking alcohol is cancer of the mouth, and the risk is irrespective of the type of drink. The risk of developing oral cancer is further increased, perhaps by up to 15 times, in those who drink alcohol and smoke compared to people who neither smoke nor drink. Both cigarette smoke and alcohol contain carcinogens, potent chemicals that are able to damage DNA and

stimulate the change from normal to cancerous in a cell. The combination of drinking and smoking is thought to be particularly damaging because the alcohol acts as a solvent, which carries the carcinogens into and through the tissues lining the mouth.

It is important to understand that oral cancer can still develop in people who neither smoke nor drink.

PREVENTION IS THE BEST POLICY

When diet, including the intake of high-sugar drinks, contributes to dental caries, the disease can be rampant, unsightly, and painful. In first teeth, dental erosion is less likely to lead to multiple tooth extraction, but when it affects the permanent teeth, erosion can be time-consuming, complex, and very expensive to treat.

Clearly, therefore, the best policy is prevention. This does not have to involve a total abstinence from alcohol and soft drinks. It is necessary simply to follow a few basic rules:

- Keep your alcohol intake within recommended guidelines: one drink a day for women and two drinks for men. If you do smoke, make a positive effort to quit.
- Opt for diet, low-sugar, sugar-free, or tooth-friendly drinks rather than their "full-sugar" counterparts.
- Moderate your intake of fruit juices and carbonated drinks. Remember also that it is better to consume these drinks reasonably quickly rather than sipping them slowly over 30 or 40 minutes.
- Never "hold" a drink in your mouth for any length of time—this can cause severe erosive damage.
- Use a straw: As long as the end of the straw is not positioned immediately behind the upper teeth but placed more toward the back of the mouth, the chance of damage to the teeth caused by either caries or erosion is reduced considerably. Some of the new generation of alcoholic drinks have high quantities of sugar, but fortunately for tooth health, there is a tendency among many consumers to drink them through a straw.

Smoking and oral health

Tobacco is as harmful for the tissues in the mouth as it is for other organs and body systems. This is true whether the tobacco is smoked as cigarettes or cigars or in a pipe—or chewed, as it is in many parts of the world.

In the United States, the prevalence of smoking reached a peak for both men and women in the 1950s and 1960s. Although the number of smokers has now fallen, approximately 25 to 30 percent of the population still smokes cigarettes on a regular basis. Most smokers are aware of the risks to general health—heart disease, stroke, high blood pressure, and cancer. The effects of smoking on oral health tend to be less well-known, although smoking commonly affects the teeth and their supporting structures and may also contribute toward the development of cancer of the mouth.

DENTAL HEALTH IN SMOKERS

There is now overwhelming evidence to suggest that the oral health of smokers is significantly worse than that of nonsmokers. In general, people who smoke have more plaque and calculus on their teeth than those who do not smoke. They also have fewer teeth. The exact reason for these observations is not known, although studies show that smokers tend to be less dentally aware and brush their teeth less often than non-smokers. This would certainly account for the lower standard of oral hygiene. The heat produced by

Smoking—an enjoyable experience?
Smoking can cause a range of problems that are socially unpleasant and indicate poor oral health. Seemingly minor mouth problems can soon become quite serious.

smoke has been shown to damage the soft tissue inside the mouth. Smokers are also at greater risk for developing gum diseases and oral cancer, although compared to other cancers, such as those of the lungs, the prevalence of mouth cancers in the West is small. Mouth cancers are much more common in parts of Asia, where chewing tobacco or paan (a mixture of chewing tobacco, betel nut, and lime paste)—as well as smoking—is popular.

What does the damage?

Cigarette smoke contains carbon monoxide, tar, and a complex cocktail of chemicals and poisons that can act either directly on the oral tissues or indirectly after being absorbed into the bloodstream. The carbon monoxide helps create an environment in which the more damaging, disease-causing bacteria are able to thrive and multiply. The tar coating the tooth surface also acts as a medium for bacteria to accumulate and leads to staining of the teeth. The chemical byproducts of smoke act directly on the soft tissues to increase the risk of leukoplakia (precancerous lesions of the tongue) and oral cancer.

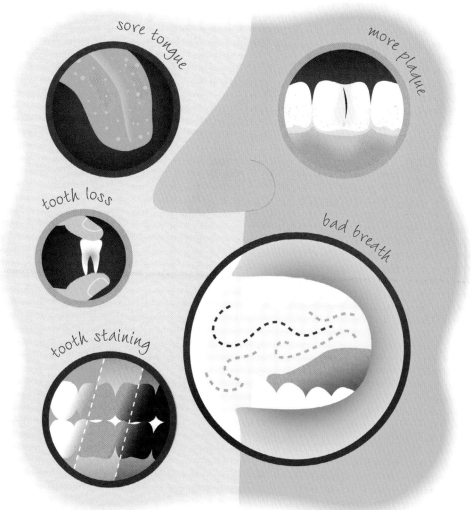

sore tongue

more plaque

tooth loss

bad breath

tooth staining

Looking for changes

The tar in tobacco causes obvious staining of the teeth that ranges from light yellow to dark brown or even black. The staining is dose-related: the more cigarettes smoked, the worse the staining. The staining is extrinsic, which means that it forms on the surface of the teeth and can therefore be removed. Staining can also affect the upper surface of the tongue, which becomes coated with a brown or black film.

Smokers' toothpastes are effective at removing stains, but they are very abrasive. If used for long periods, they may cause excessive wear on the teeth. A dentist can remove staining, but prevention is best.

Why do my gums bleed more now that I have given up smoking?

One of the most obvious symptoms of periodontal disease is bleeding gums. Nicotine, however, is a very powerful vasoconstrictor, which means that it restricts smaller blood vessels, including those in the gums. This has the effect of masking the inflamed, red appearance of periodontal disease because there is less blood flow around the tissues. Even people who have mild gum disease find that when they stop smoking their gums actually start to bleed more when they brush their teeth. A dentist can help solve this problem.

ASK THE EXPERT

Prolonged irritation from tobacco smoke results in damage to the oral mucosa and salivary glands. Smoke in the mouth causes irritation and produces heat, which can lead to chronic inflammation of the tissues of the mouth.

Sometimes, smokers might observe white patches on parts of their tongue, the roof of the mouth, or the insides of the cheeks. Thickening of the normal epithelium lining of the mouth causes these lesions, called hyperkeratosis. Occasionally, small red spots can be seen on the white lesions that occur on the roof of the mouth, but this can often resolve if smoking is stopped.

STAYING HEALTHY

Smoking and chewing tobacco increase the risk of oral cancer; this risk increases even more in those who also drink alcohol. One of the signs may be an ulcer under the tongue or in the floor of the mouth, but it is important to remember that mouth ulcers are very, very common, and in the vast majority of cases are not a cause for concern. You should have a mouth ulcer examined if
• it has been present for 2 to 3 weeks and shows no sign of healing,
• it appears to be getting bigger,
• it has a ragged edge to it, and
• it is not particularly painful.

SMOKING AND GUM DISEASES

For decades, smoking has been a recognized causal factor in a particularly painful gum infection called necrotizing ulcerative gingivitis (trench mouth), which primarily affects adolescents and young adults. This disease can be treated easily but will return if smoking is not stopped.

It is now also recognized, however, that the chemicals in cigarette smoke have a powerful effect in suppressing the inflammatory and immune systems, and, because of this, smokers tend to have more severe gum disease than do nonsmokers. This is marked by loss of tooth-supporting bone, leading to loose teeth and tooth loss. Cigarette smokers tend to be affected most, although cigar and pipe smokers are also at risk.

There is also evidence to show that for smokers who are given dental implants, there is between 10 and 30 percent more chance of losing the implants compared with nonsmokers.

Chewing tobacco increases the risk of oral cancer by five times and of tooth decay by four times.

THE BENEFITS OF QUITTING

The treatment of gum diseases in people who don't smoke is likely to be more successful than in those who do. Furthermore, after treatment, gum disease in patients who are ex-smokers tends to behave more like that of nonsmokers than smokers. This means that smoking is certainly detrimental to oral health but that quitting can help resolve gum disease, as well as offering all the other health benefits associated with not smoking.

The link between smoking and oral disease is now so clear that the training program for dentists in many parts of the United States, Canada, and the UK includes giving practical advice to patients on quitting smoking.

Stress and oral health

When stress starts to affect the body, the mouth can be one of the first areas to suffer. Stress-related mouth problems may not be serious, but they can affect confidence and self-esteem and lead to more serious conditions if not treated.

DRY MOUTH

When we experience stress, the body responds by decreasing blood flow to areas that are less important for basic survival, including the mouth. This affects salivary production and leads to dryness of the mouth. Everyone experiences a dry mouth once in a while when nervous or upset. However, chronic stress can cause a permanently dry mouth. This can be extremely uncomfortable and may lead to serious health problems.

Some of the common signs include difficulty chewing and swallowing, frequent thirst, a burning sensation of the tongue, bad breath, mouth sores, and a sore throat. If you experience persistent dry mouth, you should see your doctor or dentist, who may advise you to

- sip water or sugar-free drinks on a regular basis;
- avoid drinks with caffeine such as coffee, tea, and some soft drinks;
- chew sugar-free gum;
- avoid smoking and drinking alcohol;
- brush and floss teeth twice a day; and
- use a fluoride toothpaste.

Artificial saliva products can help with symptoms. They are available as a gel, spray, pastille, or lozenge. For advice on eating with a dry mouth, see page 87.

COLD SORES

Stress suppresses the immune system, and this can allow the herpes simplex virus (which may be dormant in the body) to spring into action, causing a cold sore blister to break out on or near the lip. Cold sores last for 7 to 14 days and can recur. Consult your pharmacist for advice on treatment.

MOUTH ULCERS

Mouth ulcers are small, painful sores that can occur anywhere in the mouth, most commonly on the inside of the cheek. They usually appear suddenly and last from 4 to 10 days. Many factors can cause mouth ulcers, but ulcers generally show that the immune system is run down or under excessive stress. The best way to avoid recurring mouth ulcers is to maintain a strong immune system by managing stress levels and eating a healthy diet with enough iron and vitamin B_{12}. Short-term relief of mouth ulcers can be gained by using a mouthwash or pastilles or by applying protective gel to the area. These can be bought over the counter, but consult your pharmacist. Some natural remedies may also be helpful:

- Rinse the mouth with a warm water and salt solution three to four times a day.
- Dab the ulcer with oil from a crushed garlic clove and hold for 30 seconds before rinsing the mouth with fresh water.
- Pierce a vitamin E capsule and apply the oil several times a day.

For severe cases, chewable steroid tablets may be prescribed. A mouth ulcer that lasts more than a few weeks should be checked by a doctor; this can be an early symptom of cancer.

HOW TO MANAGE STRESS

When stress starts to get to you, it is important to recognize it and deal with it. This can help prevent a number of mouth problems. Try the stress-busting solutions below, but see your doctor if the stress is unmanageable.

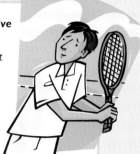

Be physically active
This may relieve the "uptight" feeling that is common with stress. Try walking, running, playing tennis, or working in the garden.

Get a good night's sleep
Make sure you get enough rest— this will improve your ability to cope with stressful situations.

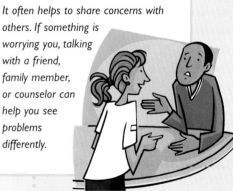

Talk to someone
It often helps to share concerns with others. If something is worrying you, talking with a friend, family member, or counselor can help you see problems differently.

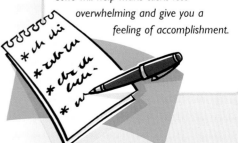

Make a list
Writing lists of things to do or remember and crossing off items when they are done will help make tasks less overwhelming and give you a feeling of accomplishment.

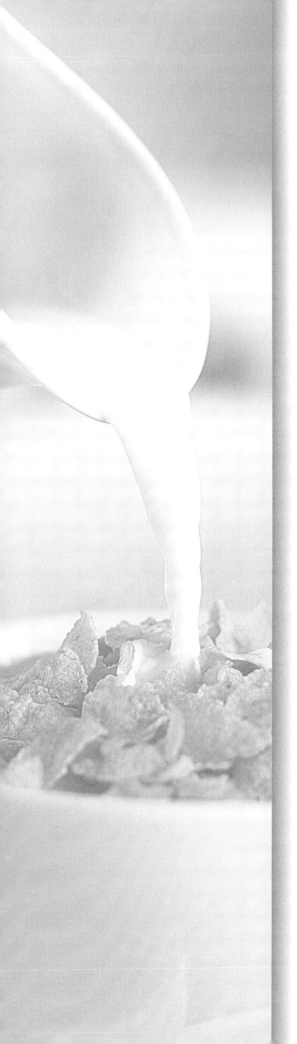

DIET AND THE EYES AND MOUTH

What and when you eat and drink has a direct impact on the health of both the eyes and mouth. Ensuring that your diet delivers the optimum daily amounts of important vitamins and minerals and avoiding the wrong food at the wrong time are steps on the road to a lifetime of visual and oral health.

79 *Vitamin A and zinc are the major nutrients your eyes need to stay healthy. Where to get them and how they work are described here.*

82 *Because diabetes can have an impact on eye health, those who suffer from this condition need to take extra care with their diet.*

83 *What you eat and drink can harm or help the teeth; advice on what to eat and what to cut down on should help preserve oral health.*

88 *Reducing sugar intake does not mean compromising on flavor. Here are some delicious recipes for low-sugar desserts.*

Eat well, see well

The foods that you eat can have a major impact on the long-term health of your eyes and how well they function, with vitamin A and the mineral zinc particularly important for good vision.

VITAL VITAMIN A

One of the functions of vitamin A is to promote good vision, especially in dim light. The chemical name for vitamin A is retinol, because it generates the pigments in the retina.

There are two forms of vitamin A in foods: retinol and carotenoids (of which beta-carotene is the most important form). Retinol can be found in foods that come from animals, such as liver and liver products; dairy products such as milk, cheese, and butter; and oily fish such as sardines, mackerel, tuna, and salmon. The richest source of retinol is marine liver oils such as those from cod, halibut, and shark, but these are usually taken in such small amounts that other foods are better dietary sources.

Carotenoids are precursors of retinol, which means that the body can make retinol from carotenoids obtained from food. Fruits and vegetables, including sweet potatoes, carrots, peppers, mangoes, dark green leafy vegetables, tomatoes, papayas, oranges, spinach, and yellow squash are the most common sources.

Retinol is the active form of vitamin A in the body. Vitamin A in foods can be expressed as retinol equivalents, basically the total amount of vitamin A in the diet derived from retinol and beta-carotene. So 1 microgram (µg) of retinol equivalent (RE) is equal to 1 microgram of retinol or 6 micrograms of beta-carotene (1 microgram is one-millionth of a gram).

Daily vitamin A requirements

A woman can obtain the daily recommended amount of vitamin A from half a pint of low-fat milk and a serving of spinach; a man might add a serving of Savoy cabbage.

The effects of deficiency

Because vitamin A is stored in the liver, it usually takes at least a year of retinol deficiency before stores become depleted. Various eye problems, including cataracts, can cause night blindness—the inability to see in dim light or at night. But night blindness may be an early sign of vitamin A deficiency. Night blindness is associated with a deficiency of a pigment called rhodopsin, or visual purple, in the light-sensitive rod cells

GOOD SOURCES OF VITAMIN A

	(OZ) PORTION	(µG) RETINOL EQUIVALENT
Calf liver, fried	3.5	25200
Lamb liver, fried	3.5	19700
Pig liver, stewed	2.5	15820
Chicken liver, fried	2.5	7350
Sweet potato, baked	1	1112
Carrots, boiled	2	756
Spinach, steamed	3	576
Red pepper, raw	2.8	512
Mango	2.8	240
Papaya	5	189
Cheese, cheddar	1.5	134
Savoy cabbage, steamed	3.4	100
Eggs, boiled	1.75	95
Tomatoes, raw	3	91
Margarine (2 tsp)	0.35	91
Butter (2 tsp)	0.35	89
Whole milk	5	81
Cod liver oil (1 tsp)	3	54
Peas, frozen	2.5	47
Apricots	1.5	36

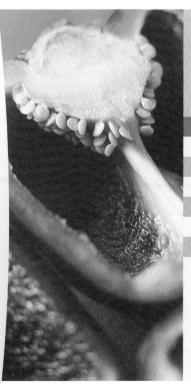

Daily vitamin A needs

The daily requirement for vitamin A in the U.S. varies according to age and gender. Adults need more than children and men need more than women.

AGE	VITAMIN A µg RE
0–6 months	420
6 months–3 years	400
4–6 years	500
7–10 years	700
11 years and older (females)	800*
11 years and older (males)	1000

* Pregnant women need an additional 200 RE a day and breast-feeding women need an additional 400 RE a day. However, pregnant women are advised not to eat liver or products containing liver, because very high levels of retinol have been associated with some birth defects.

SIX TOP FOODS FOR EYE HEALTH

1 Carrots
Full of beta-carotene, these are a prime source of vitamin A.

2 Oysters
These shellfish are the richest food source of zinc. One oyster will supply your zinc requirements for the day.

3 Oily fish
Tuna (shown here), mackerel, and salmon are all prime sources of zinc.

4 Papayas
Also called papaw or custard apple, this fruit is rich in carotenoids needed for vitamin A production.

5 Sweet potatoes
Sweet potatoes are an excellent source of the carotenoids that are converted into vitamin A.

6 Spinach
This is a good source of carotenoids, as are other green leafy vegetables such as cabbage and broccoli.

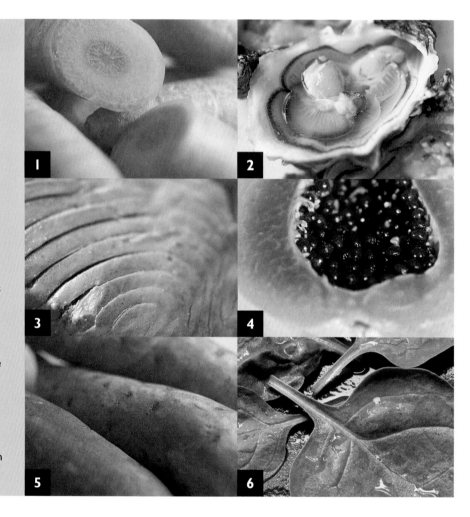

of the retina, and vitamin A is needed to form visual purple.

Manifestations of long-term vitamin A deficiency include disease in the front sections of the eye, causing xerophthalmia and keratomalacia. Xerophthalmia results from secondary infections of the surface of the eye; the conjunctiva and cornea become dry and thickened. Keratomalacia, which involves a softening of the cornea, may follow and can lead to permanent damage, resulting in blindness. Worldwide, 5 million children develop xerophthalmia every year (of whom 250,000 become blind), and many more people experience night blindness.

Carrots and night vision

Carrots contain beta-carotene, which the body converts into vitamin A. This vitamin is needed for healthy vision in dim light; deficiency can cause night blindness. Eating carrots can help ensure that you meet your daily requirement for vitamin A and thus optimize your night vision, but other foods such as liver, milk, cheese, dark green leafy vegetables, and eggs also supply this vitamin and are equally significant in combating vitamin A deficiency.

THE IMPORTANCE OF ZINC

Zinc is needed to form an enzyme called retinol dehydrogenase, which helps vitamin A work in the eye. Prime sources include:

- **Oysters** There are 71 milligrams of zinc in six raw oysters. Other shellfish are also good zinc sources.
- **Beef** Five ounces of stewed braising steak supplies 13.3 milligrams of zinc.
- **Pork, lamb and chicken** A lamb chop has about 3 milligrams of zinc, a serving of roast chicken averages 2.2 milligrams of zinc; and two slices of ham gives you 1 milligram of zinc.
- **Pecans and pumpkin seeds** A handful of pecans contains 3.2 milligrams of zinc, and a tablespoon of pumpkin seeds has 1.1 milligrams of zinc.

Other good food sources that contain as much as 1 milligram of zinc in an average portion are cheese, fish, liver, kidney, eggs, and potatoes. There is about 0.5 milligram of zinc in two slices of bread (brown bread contains more zinc than white) or 5 ounces of whole milk.

Daily zinc needs

The daily recommended amount of zinc is 15 milligrams for adults. This can be achieved by eating a serving of steak or one oyster. Alternatively, an adult could cover his or her daily zinc requirement by eating a boiled egg, four slices of brown bread, a serving of cheddar cheese, a handful of pecans, and a lamb chop.

SUPPLEMENTS AND AMD

There have been suggestions that taking antioxidant vitamin and mineral supplements such as zinc and vitamins A, C, and E may slow down the progression of age-related macular degeneration (AMD; see page 134) by taking up the free radicals (produced in the process of absorbing light) that damage the macula. Evidence indicates that supplements are effective in halting the progression of AMD in people with moderate or severe signs of the disease. There is no convincing evidence, however, to suggest that people with early signs of AMD should take supplements; indeed, long-term supplementation can be harmful, particularly for smokers, for whom the risk of heart disease and of lung cancer are increased.

Some studies have indicated that people who maintain a diet rich in antioxidant vitamins and minerals such as carotenoids, vitamins C and E, selenium, and zinc may be less

Why does chopping onions make the eyes water?

TALKING POINT

When you chop an onion, you break open some of its cells. This releases enzymes that in turn break down a compound called allicin in the onion to make a substance called propenyl sulfuric acid. This fumes up from the onion and, because it is an irritant, our eyes automatically blink and produce water in an attempt to flush away the sulfuric acid. A reflex action to get rid of a foreign substance in the eyes is to rub them with our hands; when chopping onions, this only makes the situation worse because the hands are already covered with sulfuric acid from cutting the onion. Ways to alleviate the problem include

- Chilling onions for 20 minutes before chopping them; this slows down the reaction between allicin and the enzyme.
- Cutting the onions under cold running water.
- Slicing rather than chopping onions to minimize the number of onion cells that are crushed, so less sulfuric acid is produced.
- Wearing goggles to prevent the fumes from reaching your eyes.

likely to develop AMD. Trials have failed to show that taking antioxidant supplements prevents or delays the onset of AMD.

Lutein supplements

Lutein and zeaxanthin are yellow pigments in the macula that help protect it from damage by free radicals. AMD patients have low levels of these pigments, so lutein in particular is sold as a dietary supplement. However, there is no evidence as yet that lutein supplements effectively combat AMD or

even that taking them increases lutein levels in the macula.

Bilberries and the eyes
Bilberries (similar to blueberries) are rich in compounds called anthocyanosides, which speed up regeneration of rhodopsin—a pigment needed for vision in dim light. Research suggests that bilberries can improve adaptation to the dark in people with poor vision but not in people with healthy vision.

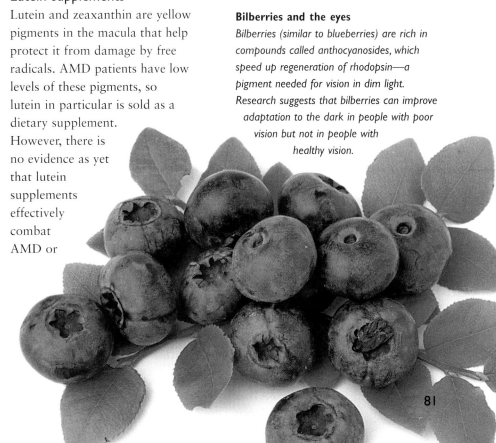

Eye health and diabetes

Diabetics are particularly susceptible to eye damage. Deterioration of the retina is common, especially among those who have had diabetes for a long time, and it is the most frequent cause of blindness among diabetics below age 65.

THE RISK OF EYE DAMAGE

Diabetes mellitus is a chronic illness that affects about 10 million people in the United States and about 110 million worldwide. In addition to carrying a high risk to the condition of the eyes, diabetes increases the risks of heart and kidney disease and damage to the nerves and limbs.

Diabetic retinopathy (see page 137) occurs when diabetes affects the retina, causing blood vessels in the retina to leak and affect the eye's ability to function properly. The severity of retinopathy may differ in each eye. It is estimated that one in every two people with diabetes has some degree of retinopathy.

FOOD SENSE FOR DIABETICS

Eating well and paying attention to diet is one of the most important ways for anyone with diabetes to reduce the chance of developing diabetic retinopathy or any other complication associated with diabetes. Also very important are controlling blood pressure and blood sugar levels, maintaining a sensible weight, exercising, and not smoking.

Contrary to popular belief, people with diabetes can enjoy the same foods as everyone else, including those containing sugar, but their diet must be balanced and more care has to be taken with the timing of meals and snacks. The advice of a dietitian is often helpful and can be essential.

Starchy foods

It is best if the quantity and timing of eating starchy foods remain constant from day to day. Whole-meal or whole-grain starchy foods are higher in fiber, which will help keep the GI tract healthy and also fill you up.

Fruit and vegetables

Fresh, frozen, canned, and dried fruit and vegetables all count toward the goal of at least five servings a day.

Cut down on fat

Buy low- or reduced-fat dairy products. Choose lean meats whenever possible, and trim off excess fat or skin. Avoid frying as a cooking method. Reduce the amount of fat used on bread and potatoes or in cooking. Use monounsaturated oils such as olive or rapeseed rather than saturated fats such as butter and lard.

Keep sugary foods to a minimum

Choose sugar-free, low-sugar, or "diet" soft drinks. Use artificial sweeteners such as saccharin or aspartame instead of sugar. Choose high-fiber, low-sugar cookies and cakes.

Use less salt (sodium chloride)

Keep in mind that most processed foods contain sodium This includes bread, cereals, ham, bacon, cheese, cookies, canned foods, packaged soups, bouillon cubes, and yeast extract. Flavor foods with herbs, spices, or lemon juice or use low-sodium salt substitutes or soy sauce.

Consume alcohol in moderation

Women with diabetes should drink no more than one drink a day and men no more than two. Examples of a unit are one small glass of wine or 12 ounces of beer.

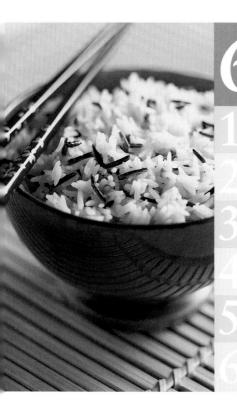

6 TIPS TO HELP DIABETICS

The American Diabetes Association recommends that people with diabetes should:

1. Make sure to eat foods from all food groups every day. Carbohydrates (for energy) and protein (for growth and energy) are particularly important.

2. Make sure to maintain adequate fiber intake. Fiber may help lower blood glucose and blood fat levels.

3. Reduce fat intake, particularly saturated (animal) fat, to maintain a healthy body weight and reduce the risk of heart disease as well as diabetes complications.

4. Limit sugar intake. Sugar in food and drinks can encourage the level of glucose in the blood to rise too quickly.

5. Use less salt. Reducing salt lowers blood pressure and therefore is helpful in guarding against diabetic retinopathy.

6. Drink alcohol only in moderation. Don't drink alcohol on an empty stomach because this can help cause glucose levels in the blood to drop too low.

Diet and oral health

There is a lot that individuals can do to preserve the health of their teeth through diet, both by limiting the intake of certain foods and ensuring adequate dietary amounts of others. Eating and tooth brushing at the right time also help.

HOW FOOD AFFECTS THE TEETH

Plaque on the surface of the teeth contains bacteria that make acids by fermenting sugars from foods or as a result of the breakdown of carbohydrates during digestion. Acid production lowers the pH of the surface of the tooth. When the pH drops to about 5.5, demineralization occurs—that is, calcium and phosphate dissolve. Saliva in the mouth gradually helps neutralize these acids and bring the pH back up above 5.5, thereby helping the dissolved calcium and phosphate return to the tooth enamel. This process is known as remineralization.

If food and drink containing sugar and carbohydrates are nibbled throughout the day, there may not be enough time between eating or drinking episodes for remineralization to occur (see page 60). A time period of 2 to 3 hours between sugar intakes is required to allow remineralization to occur so the teeth can repair themselves. Over a period of time, if demineralization is greater than remineralization, tooth decay will result.

PROTECTING THE TEETH

Some foods may actually help protect against the development of tooth decay.

- Substances called phosphates attach themselves to the tooth surface and thus reduce the amount of enamel that is dissolved. The most effective phosphate is contained in compounds called phytates, which are found in grains, seeds, cereals, vegetables, and fruits. The disadvantage of phytates is that they reduce the body's absorption of minerals such as iron and zinc, so a balance is important.
- Foods high in fiber (such as whole-grain cereals, fruits, and vegetables) may help increase the flow of saliva in the mouth, thereby raising pH levels.
- Milk, cheese, and natural yogurt have the ability to raise the pH in the mouth and so help reduce the exposure of teeth to acids. They also contain high levels of calcium and phosphate, as well as casein and other proteins that are absorbed onto the surface of the enamel. Both of these factors prevent the enamel from dissolving.

SUGARS AND TOOTH DECAY

Although all sugars and carbohydrates are absorbed by the body to provide energy, they have a range of different effects within the body. Eating certain types of sugary foods and drinks at frequent intervals—and especially between meals—has been linked with increased tooth decay. According to studies done on the effects of sugar on teeth, the type of sugar and where it is located in the food affects its

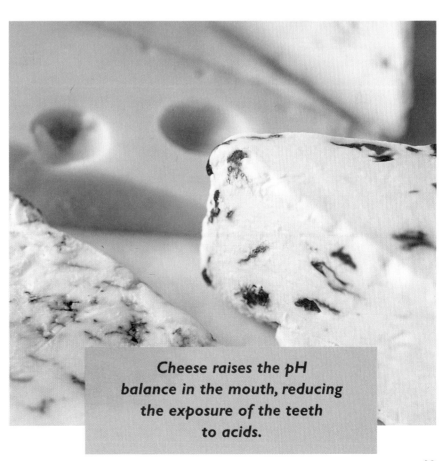

Cheese raises the pH balance in the mouth, reducing the exposure of the teeth to acids.

likelihood of causing decay. Sugars are therefore classified as intrinsic or extrinsic.

- Intrinsic sugars are those contained in the cells of foods, such as those from whole fruits and vegetables.
- Extrinsic sugars are those not contained in the cells of foods, such as milk sugars (found in milk and milk products) and sugars in fruit juices, table sugar, and sugars added to foods.

It is generally thought that intrinsic sugars—and milk sugars, which are extrinsic—do not have adverse effects on the teeth, whereas other extrinsic sugars play a part in dental decay.

Fresh fruit is not strongly linked with tooth decay. This is thought to be true because sugars in fruit are held in the cells of the fruit and aren't released until chewing breaks down the cells. They also contain fiber; this stimulates the production of saliva, which "cleanses" the mouth.

Sweetened fruit juices, however, are thought to be more cariogenic (causing tooth decay); this is thought to result from the added sugars.

Sticky or not sticky?

Another factor that affects the likelihood of developing tooth decay is the stickiness of the food we eat. Toffee, cotton candy, and nougat, for example, can stick to the teeth and thus may lower the pH in the mouth for a longer period of time.

Sweets or chocolate?

There is some research to suggest that chocolate may be less cariogenic than other sweets, even if it is eaten frequently and between meals. Animal experiments have suggested that chocolate contains caries-protective factors such as cocoa. It is also less sticky than some sweets and therefore tends to be in contact with the teeth for a shorter time.

Hidden sources of sugars

Many sweet and tasty foods and drinks contain sugar. Sugar comes in various forms, some of which do not automatically sound as if they are sugar. Names to look for when reading the ingredients list on food labels include

Three quarters of our sugar intake comes from junk foods and sweets.

- Sucrose This is the product we know as "sugar," found in cakes and cookies.
- Dextrose This is a natural form of glucose found in grains, vegetables, and legumes. It is healthier than the artifical glucose in sports drinks.
- Fructose This is the sweetest of all sugars. It occurs naturally in honey and fruits.
- Lactose This sugar is found in milk and dairy products. It is about a third as sweet as sucrose.

ACID EROSION

Some fruit juices and fruits such as oranges, lemons, and limes can cause dental erosion. This is not the same as tooth decay; it results from the gradual loss of enamel from the tooth. In children and adolescents, acidic soft drinks are the main cause of erosion. A study of adult patients by dentists in Finland showed the following list of foods in order of risk: citrus fruits, other fruits, soft drinks, sports drinks, pickles, and cider vinegar.

Acid drinks consumed before bed cause the most damage because the production of saliva is low during the night, so the acid continues to demineralize the teeth for a much longer period of time. You can reduce the contact of acidic drinks and your teeth by drinking through a straw rather than from a glass.

Timing tooth brushing

Contrary to the traditional advice to brush your teeth after a meal, tooth brushing should not

---

ON THE CUTTING EDGE

Modified lactobacilli may prevent cavities

Research by a team of scientists from Sweden, Britain, and Holland has shown that a certain type of bacteria may help in the prevention of tooth decay.

The main culprit in decay has been identified as a strain of bacteria called *Streptococcus mutans*. This bacterium ferments sugars and starches, which results in acid being produced within minutes of being exposed. The group of researchers has been able to develop a cavity-friendly strain of bacteria called lactobacillus, which helps reduce the number of *S. mutans*. Tests with rats have shown that the friendly bacteria reduced the number of *S. mutans* bacteria in the rats' mouths and also reduced the number of cavities in their teeth.

The lactobacillus strain stayed in the mouth for 3 weeks, continually fighting the streptococci and preventing dental decay.

MENU *IMPORTANCE OF CALCIUM*

Calcium helps keep teeth strong and healthy. The main sources of calcium in the average American diet are dairy products such as milk, yogurt, and cheese and leafy green vegetables. Many breads in the U.S. are fortified with calcium, and hard water and fish with bones such as canned sardines and salmon are also important sources. The average daily requirement for calcium for adults is 1000 milligrams a day.

breakfast

- 1½ oz bran muffin, glass of calcium-fortified orange juice, cup of fruit tea = 424 mg calcium (50 + 325 + 49)
- large boiled egg, 2 slices whole-grain toast with low-fat spread, cup of tea = 116 mg calcium (29 + 38 + 49)

lunch

- 3.5 oz sardines grilled with handful of sesame seeds until seeds have toasted, served with medley of cauliflower and broccoli = 593 mg calcium (540 + 25 + 28)
- 4¾ oz baked beans on toast, followed by container of yogurt = 403 mg calcium (65 + 38 + 300)

dinner

- 3 oz roast chicken, served with a baked potato topped with 1¾ oz plain yogurt, mixed leaf salad of watercress and baby spinach = 293 mg calcium (110 + 100 + 83)
- 8¾ oz mixed bean stew, served with 4.5 oz boiled rice, date, and orange salad = 134 mg calcium (90 + 12 + 6 + 26)

snacks and drinks

- 1¼ cup skim milk = 350 mg calcium
- 1¼ cup fortified soy milk = 300 mg calcium
- 4.5 oz sesame seeds = 100 mg calcium
- 1.5 oz (handful) dry roasted peanuts = 21 mg calcium
- ¾ oz (1 tbsp) raisins = 12 mg calcium
- 6 oz (1 medium) banana = 10 mg calcium
- 3.5 oz (1 medium) apple = 4 mg calcium

HIGH CALCIUM, LOW FAT

Many of the best sources of calcium are dairy products, which can be high in fat and harmful to weight control and to the heart, so choose low-fat or fat-free versions when possible. A food is considered high in calcium if it provides at least 250 mg in an average serving. Such foods include low-fat yogurt, low-fat milk, and cottage cheese. Nonfat dried milk can also be added to foods like mashed potatoes, cereals, and soups to improve their calcium content.

---

be encouraged immediately after eating acidic foods or drinks. When acids and teeth make contact, the tooth enamel begins to lose calcium. This process is reversed if you leave enough time for saliva to be produced and remineralization to take place, but if people brush their teeth immediately after consuming the food or drink, the enamel may be removed.

DIET AND CHILDREN'S TEETH

The first teeth erupt at around 6 months of age, and avoiding the unnecessary consumption of extrinsic sugars should ensure sensible dietary habits from early in life.

Fruit juices or baby drinks can be given after the age of 6 months, but because these drinks contain high levels of acids, they should always be diluted to at least one part of juice to five parts of water and given only at mealtimes. For tooth health, only water and milk should be given as drinks between meals.

Extensive dental caries have been linked to infants and children being given bottles containing sweetened drinks and pacifiers sweetened with honey or jam.

FOOD AND THE GUMS

Gingivitis, or inflammation of the gums, usually occurs as a result of infection from food debris that gets stuck in the gaps at the bottom of the teeth. Continued inflammation of the gums can result in the gums pulling away from the teeth, allowing the formation of "pockets" filled with bacterial plaque, calculus, and food debris. Periodontal disease then develops, leading to bone loss around the teeth and, as a result, the teeth become loose and fall out. Drinking water after meals can help dislodge and remove food particles, as will regular flossing.

EATING AND DRINKING HABITS FOR HEALTHY TEETH

There are several ways to protect against dental disease, all of which combine for best effect.

- Reduce the consumption and frequency of foods and drinks containing sugar, being careful to avoid sticky or chewy foods, which should not be eaten between meals.
- Finish off a meal with a piece of cheese or a glass of milk.
- Don't brush your teeth right after drinking acidic liquids.
- Leave 1 to 2 hours between eating or drinking and brushing to allow saliva to neutralize acids and for remineralization to occur.
- Drink water, milk, or tea between meals, because these are not acidic.
- Avoid acidic or sugary drinks, such as hot chocolate, last thing at night. Drink water instead.

Vitamin D

Vitamin D helps the body absorb calcium from food. Vitamin D is made through the action of sunlight on a substance in the skin; this is the most important source for most people.

The main sources of vitamin D in the diet are meat, margarine, oily fish, fortified breakfast cereals, and eggs. In the United States, margarine is fortified with vitamin D, and many reduced-fat spreads are also fortified.

Most people obtain sufficient vitamin D from sunlight, so there isn't a recommended daily dietary requirement for adults. However, pregnant and breast-feeding women, the elderly, and children up to 5 years old have specific requirements that may require the use of dietary supplements, such as cod liver oil. Pregnant and lactating women and the elderly require 10 micrograms a day, and children between the ages of 1 and 4 years old need 7 micrograms a day.

FOODS AND DRINKS FOR ORAL HEALTH

- **Cheese** Finish off a meal with a piece of cheese—if you are watching your weight, choose one naturally lower in fat, such as Edam.
- **Milk** Drink milk between meals and choose skim or low-fat milk to keep the fat levels down. Try it ice cold from the fridge.
- **Tea** Drink it between meals—green, black, and herbal are all beneficial.
- **Water** The cheapest drink in town, it has no calories and plenty of minerals to keep teeth healthy.
- **Fruits and vegetables** These contain antioxidants, which protect gums from cell damage.

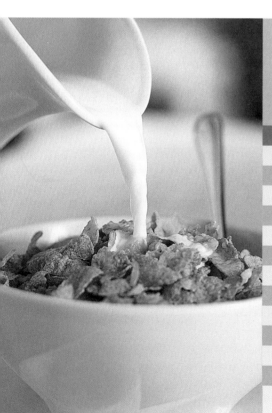

Vitamin D content of selected foods

The major function of vitamin D is to promote the absorption of calcium. Few foods are naturally rich in vitamin D—most people get enough from exposure to sunlight. However, season, latitude, time of day, cloud cover, and the use of suncreen all affect exposure to sunlight, making it important to include good sources of vitamin D in your diet.

	PORTION (oz)	VITAMIN D (µg)
Salmon, canned	4.2, 1 serving	20.6
Herring, grilled	4.2, 1 serving	19.2
Salmon, grilled	2.8, medium fillet	7.9
Cod liver oil	0.1, 1 tsp	6.3
Beef, braised	5, 1 serving	1.1
Pork loin chop, grilled	4.2, 1 chop	1
Egg, boiled	1.75, 1 egg	0.9
Margarine	0.35, 2 tsp	0.8
Cornflakes	1, 1 bowl	0.6
Lamb chop, grilled	2.5, 1 chop	0.4
Chicken drumstick, roasted	3.5, 1 large	0.1
Chicken breast, grilled	4.5, 1 large	0.1
Cheddar cheese	1.4, small chunk	0.1

PROTECTIVE FLUORIDE

Fluoride is a useful mineral that is incorporated into teeth as they form. It can reduce dental caries by 30 to 50 percent and makes the enamel less soluble to acid. Fluoride also reduces acid production by plaque bacteria and enhances the remineralization process.

In some parts of the country, fluoride is naturally present in drinking water. If the fluoride content is low, it may be added by the local water company. The optimal amount of fluoride is 1 part per million.

However, excessive fluoride intake during childhood can cause dental fluorosis, which is the discoloration of tooth enamel that occurs as the teeth develop. In mild cases, the teeth may have chalky white patches; in severe cases, they may have dark brown stains—these effects are irreversible. The amount of fluoride in fluoride toothpastes and mouth rinses is very high. Children should only use a pea-sized amount of child-formula toothpaste and be taught not to swallow toothpaste.

HARD-WORKING SALIVA

Saliva helps protect teeth from dental caries by:
- helping wash pieces of food away from the teeth;
- neutralizing acids produced by bacteria;
- carrying minerals such as calcium, phosphate, and fluoride to the tooth surface, which helps remineralization; and
- preventing dry mouth, which creates an ideal environment for caries-causing bacteria.

Artificial saliva products can help in cases of xerostomia (see page 155).

EATING WITH A DRY MOUTH

A dry mouth can make eating difficult, even painful, particularly dry and "thick" foods such as chips, cookies, and crackers. However, some foods and drinks can be helpful:
- Eat pineapple chunks, yogurt, ice cubes, and frozen tonic water.
- Have sauces and gravy with meals.
- Keep the mouth moist by drinking water throughout the day. Rinse the mouth with 1 teaspoon of vegetable oil or some softened butter at night.
- Include foods with a high water content, such as jelly.
- Drink fluids with your meals.

BAD BREATH, FOOD, AND DRINK

Some foods and drinks can temporarily cause bad breath, or halitosis. The major culprits include
- spicy foods, the odors of which can last for hours;
- cheese such as blue cheese, Camembert, or Roquefort;
- onions and garlic;
- tuna;
- wine, beer, and whisky; and
- coffee.

During fasting or starvation, the body's store of glycogen (a form of carbohydrate that releases fuel for the body to use) is depleted. In order to keep a supply of fuel for the body to function properly, protein has to be broken down to make fuel, and during this process compounds called ketones are produced. Ketones make the breath smell bad.

There are, however, other causes of bad breath not directly related to food, such as stress (see page 77). Conditions such as tonsillitis, constipation, indigestion, ulcers, infected gums, bronchitis, and catarrh can also cause bad breath.

Herbs for oral health
Some herbs have been suggested by herbalists and naturopaths as being able to cleanse the mouth, freshen breath, and ease tooth pain.

Parsley *has been chewed since Roman times to counter mouth odors; parsley oil is still used in breath fresheners.*

Alfalfa *is rich in chorophyll, which has a deodorizing effect. Try alfalfa "tea" several times a day.*

Cloves *have long been used to ease toothache, especially as oil of cloves.* Ginger *may also ease toothache, and* cinnamon *has a similar but milder effect.*

Goldenseal *extract eases mouth sores or infected gums.* Dill seeds *can prevent bad breath.*

Peppermint, rosemary, cloves, and fennel *can all help freshen the breath.*

87

Low-sugar, high-flavor desserts

Cutting down on your sugar intake to protect your teeth does not have to be difficult—most fruits are rich in natural sugars and full of flavor. If you do not want to give up on sweets, try these delicious desserts.

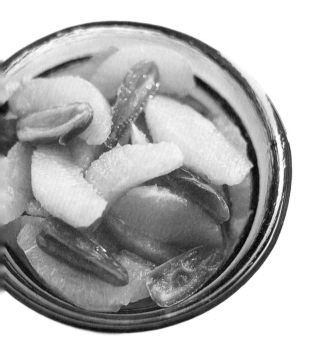

LUSCIOUS MELONS WITH CHEESE

1 large yellow
   cantaloupe
1 tbsp raspberry liqueur
5½ oz Gorgonzola cheese
Handful of chopped mint

Either slice the melon and cut it into cubes or make melon balls. Place the cubes or balls in a large serving bowl and drizzle over the raspberry cordial. Crumble the Gorgonzola cheese over the top and sprinkle with chopped mint. Chill before serving.
Serves 4

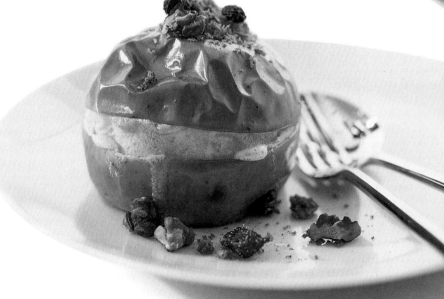

ORANGE AND DATE SALAD

6 large oranges
6 large dates, pitted and chopped
1 carton of ruby-red grapefruit juice
1 tbsp elderflower liqueur

Peel the oranges, cut them into thick slices, and place in a large serving bowl. Add the chopped dates and mix, then pour over the grapefruit juice and elderflower liqueur. Let the mixture infuse in the refrigerator for at least 30 minutes before serving.
Serves 4–6

STUFFED BAKED APPLES

4 cooking apples
1¾ oz brown breadcrumbs
1¾ oz chopped walnuts
1¾ oz raisins
½ tsp ground cinnamon
Grated peel from ½ lemon

Core the apples, slit them around the middle, and set aside. Mix the remaining ingredients together and use to stuff the apples. Place mixture in a baking dish and bake in a moderate oven (350°F) for about 45–55 minutes, or until soft.
Serves 4

BANANA BOATS

4 large bananas
8-oz mascarpone cheese

Peel the bananas and wrap them individually in foil. Bake in a moderate oven (350°F) for 10–15 minutes. Unfold the foil and top with mascarpone. Remove the foil from the bananas just before eating.
Serves 4

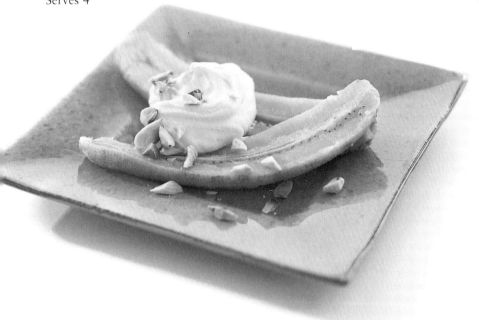

COMPOTE OF SPICED DRIED FRUITS

1 large mug of Earl Grey tea
4½ oz dried apricots
3½ oz raisins
3½ oz dried figs
3½ oz dried cranberries
1 cinnamon stick
1 slice of fresh ginger
Grated zest of 1 lime

Put the tea in a saucepan and bring to a boil. Add the remaining ingredients and simmer for 15 minutes. Leave to cool slightly before serving.
Serves 4–6

MEDITERRANEAN SWEET COUSCOUS

14 oz couscous
About 2 cups hot water
1 tbsp orange blossom water
6 large ready-to-eat dried apricots cut into quarters
Large handful toasted almonds
Large handful toasted pistachio nuts
6 figs cut into halves
3 small containers of low-fat yogurt

Place the couscous in a large serving bowl, pour over enough hot water to cover (about 2 cups), add the orange blossom water, and cover with a plate or plastic wrap. Leave for about 10 minutes until all the water has been absorbed. Fluff up the grains of couscous with a fork. Add the dried apricots and mixed nuts and mix thoroughly, then top with the halved figs. Serve with the yogurt.
Serves 4

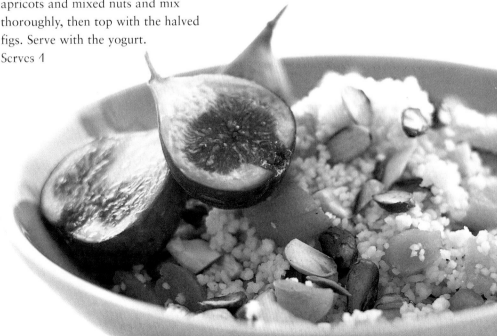

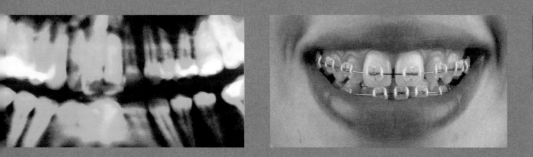
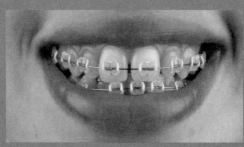
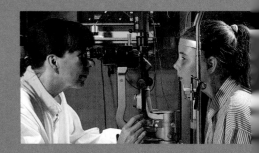

3

What happens
when things go wrong

Knowing what can go wrong with eyes

Problems with eyes and vision fall into two categories: those related to the focusing system of the eye and those related to eye health. Focusing disorders are rarely a cause for concern and can be corrected easily. Eye health problems, in contrast, may be more serious and difficult to treat.

Some health problems can be picked up in a routine eye examination by an optometrist (who will then refer patients to a physician), which is why it is important to have regular eye checkups, whether or not there has been a detectable change in eyesight.

FOCUSING PROBLEMS

Only a minority of us have perfect vision. Genes and lifestyle both contribute to determining who will need eyeglasses. There are three very common types of focusing problems, also known as "refractive error." These are nearsightedness (myopia), farsightedness (hypermetropia), and astigmatism. Two other common conditions are amblyopia (sometimes called a "lazy" eye) and presbyopia (the deterioration of near vision in middle age).

- **Nearsightedness (myopia)** In myopia, objects in the distance cannot be seen clearly because the refractive system of the eye bends light from a distant object too much, bringing it to a focus in front of rather than on the retina. Myopia is usually the result of the eyeball being slightly elongated.
- **Farsightedness (hypermetropia)** Objects close to the eye are blurred. This is because the refractive system of the eye bends light from close objects too little, failing to bring it to a focus before the light reaches the retina. Hypermetropia is usually inherited and is generally the result of the eyeball being too short.
- **Astigmatism** In this usually inherited condition, the cornea—which ideally should be evenly curved like a soccer ball—is actually shaped more like a football.

Light entering the eye through different parts of the cornea is brought in focus at different points, with the result that vision is blurred and distorted.
- **Amblyopia (lazy eye)** Amblyopia first begins in childhood and can be the result of either a big difference in the focusing ability of the two eyes or a squint, in which the movement of the eyes is poorly coordinated. The brain gradually learns to ignore the image received from one of the eyes, and a failure to treat the underlying problem

Threats to eye health
Some major eye problems are listed below together with, where applicable, the U.S. incidence rate.

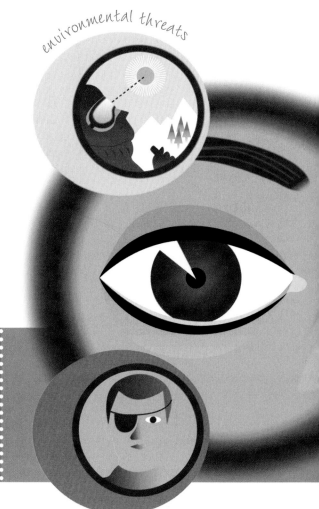

environmental threats

trauma

MORE COMMON

SERIOUS VISUAL DISABILITY AND BLINDNESS	AGE-RELATED MACULAR DEGENERATION
100 million Americans are visually disabled without corrective lenses; 70 million of them are myopic. 1.1 million are legally blind	*13 million people have signs of macular degeneration; 1.2 million are in the later stages of it, and 230,000 are blind from it.*

in childhood can result in poor "stereo" vision and depth perception for the rest of a patient's life.

- **Presbyopia** Development of the eye continues through life. People in their 40s notice a gradual change in vision, often characterized by a need to hold reading material further away from the eyes. This effect—known as presbyopia—happens to everyone and is caused by changes in the flexibility and shape of the lens. In order to focus on the retina, light from close objects must be bent more than light from distant objects. The maximum power of the eye's lens slowly decreases with age, so you are less able to focus on close objects.

AGE-RELATED DISEASES AND DISORDERS

The brain's ability to compensate for certain visual problems means that serious eye conditions can develop without obvious symptoms, and a regular eye checkup is important even if you believe your vision to be good. The leading causes of blindness in the U.S. are age-related macular degeneration, glaucoma, diabetic retinopathy,

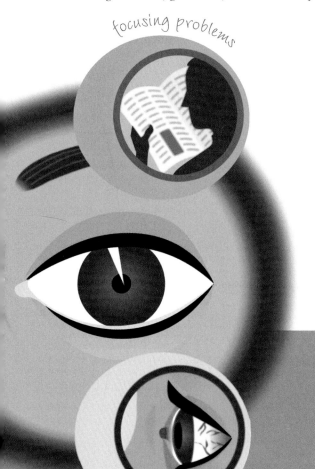

focusing problems

infections

Does close work cause myopia?

Myopia tends to run in families, and eye strain from close work during childhood, such as reading, is thought by some to encourage its development. It has been suggested that leaving lights on in children's bedrooms at night leads to myopia, but this has not been supported by research. Turning the light off in a child's bedroom may not be a good idea either; this may encourage the child to read in poor light, using a flashlight, for example. It is always best to read in good light.

ASK THE EXPERT

and cataracts. All are linked to the aging process, and become more common and severe with increasing age.

- **Age-related macular degeneration** AMD is characterized by a wasting of the central part of the retina. The cause is unknown, although research has suggested that a diet rich in antioxidants may reduce the risk of developing the condition. AMD produces distortion and eventually a loss of the central part of the vision (see page 134).
- **Glaucoma** The most common form of glaucoma is a progressive long-term condition that generally affects people over 40, in which a gradual buildup of pressure of the fluid inside the eye slowly damages the optic nerve. In the chronic form of glaucoma (see page 139), there are no symptoms until damage has become severe, when a loss of side vision is noticed. Early detection is vital to successful treatment.
- **Diabetic retinopathy** Diabetes can cause blood vessels supplying the retina to leak and damage the retina. Fluid leaking into the retina interferes with its function and, in severe cases, scar tissue can form, which increases the risk of retinal detachment (see page 144).

LESS COMMON

GLAUCOMA
2 million people are visually impaired by glaucoma; 1 million more don't know they have the disease. 5,000 people become blind each year because of glaucoma.

CATARACTS
5.5 million people have vision obstructed by cataracts; there are 400,000 new cases each year.

DIABETIC RETINOPATHY
Between 600,000 and 700,000 Americans have diabetic retinopathy severe enough to cause vision loss; 24,000 go blind annually.

- **Cataracts** A cataract is a loss of transparency in the lens of the eye, causing misty or blurred vision (see page 135). By far the most common cause is aging. Other causes include injury, diseases such as diabetes, certain drugs, and radiation, notably UV rays from the sun.

NERVE DAMAGE

There is more to vision than a transparent lens and a healthy retina. Visual problems such as blind spots can arise from nerve damage, as from a stroke or brain tumor. Damage may disrupt messages traveling along nerves from the eye to the brain or the interpretation of those messages in the brain. Similarly, damage to nerves controlling the muscles of eye movement can cause a squint, in which coordination of eye movement is faulty.

CANCER

Ocular tumors are rare but potentially fatal (see page 110). In the past, the solution was to remove the affected eye, but today there are often other options including radiation and laser treatments.

COLOR BLINDNESS

This is usually caused by an inherited lack of one or more of the color receptors in the retina. It can also occur as the result of disease. It is very rare for someone who is called "color blind" to have no color perception at all. It is far more common for such a person to have difficulty distinguishing two colors—usually red and green. Inherited color blindness is much more common in boys than in girls.

INFECTION

The body's first line of defense against environmental threats lies in its external surfaces. The front surface of

Eyesight and increasing age
Most people find that at some point they begin to need glasses to see objects clearly at close range, and chances are that some will develop a more complex eye disorder. However, the choice of treatments for many age-related conditions, ranging from corrective lenses to surgical intervention, has never been greater.

the eye is therefore a potential site of attack by infectious agents and chemicals—pollutants and allergens—causing symptoms such as pain, itchiness, watering, redness, and puffiness. Some infections are innocuous, but others can cause sight-threatening scarring on the cornea or tissue damage inside the eye. Infections often reach the eye through hand-eye contact. For contact lens wearers, particles trapped behind a lens can enable infectious agents to enter the eye. Tap water must not be used to clean lenses, because it may contain an infectious organism called Acanthamoeba, which can cause corneal ulcers.

TRAUMA

Accidents to the eye are commonplace and can occur at home, at work, and while playing sports. Eye-protecting, shatterproof goggles and eye shields are a health and safety requirement for many jobs on factory floors and in workshops (see page 64).

ULTRAVIOLET RADIATION

Ultraviolet (UV) radiation in sunlight can trigger snow blindness and over the long term encourages the development of cataracts. People who spend long periods outside, at work or for leisure, should consider eyewear with built-in UV protection—particularly in bright, reflective conditions such as around water or snow. There is no convincing evidence that radiation from computer screens causes eye problems.

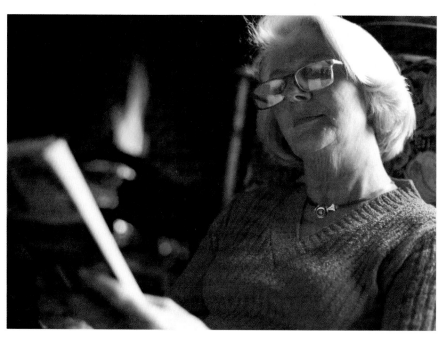

Who's who—meet the eye specialists

Who does what in the world of eye care can be confusing. The experts you are most likely to meet are the ophthalmic optician (optometrist), the dispensing optician, and the ophthalmologist.

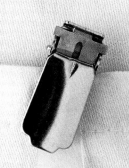

OPHTHALMIC OPTICIAN/OPTOMETRIST

An ophthalmic optician—also called an optometrist—conducts tests to measure how well you can see and prescribes glasses or contact lenses to correct disorders of vision such as near- or farsightedness. An optometrist will also give advice on the best types of glasses or contact lenses for your eyes and vision requirements. In addition, an optometrist will examine your eyes externally and internally in order to check for any signs of eye diseases or abnormalities.

DISPENSING OPTICIAN

A dispensing optician fills written prescriptions (from optometrists or ophthalmologists) and recommends frames and lenses best suited to the wearer's prescription, visual requirements, and facial features. With these considerations in mind, a dispensing optician prepares the work order that provides the information needed to grind and insert lenses into a frame. Some do this themselves, although technicians often carry out this part of the job. Dispensing opticians will advise a patient on wearing and caring for glasses and can also fix broken frames. Some specialize in fitting contact lenses.

PHYSICIAN

The family doctor, although not an expert in eye care, still has an important role to play in this area. If a physician notices signs of a vision problem, he or she will recommend that the patient have vision tests. An optometrist who spots signs that require additional investigation and, possibly, medical attention, will refer the patient to his or her physician, who then manages any medical treatment or, if necessary, coordinates the referral of the patient to the appropriate specialist.

ORTHOPTIST

An orthoptist is a specialist in the muscles of the eye. Orthoptists undergo professional training to become

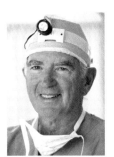

OPHTHALMOLOGIST

An ophthalmologist is a medical doctor who has specialized in eye diseases and disorders of the visual system (ophthalmology). Ophthalmologists are trained to diagnose and manage all eye problems, although they often have their own specialty areas. Most perform surgery for problems such as cataracts, squints, diabetic eye disease, refractive errors, and corneal disease. They work in hospitals and private clinics.

experts in problems of eye movement, eye alignment, and disorders of vision in children and adults. They usually work under an ophthalmologist as part of a team assessing patients who have been referred to the ophthalmologist. Orthoptists evaluate vision, measure eye position, and participate in patient education and treatment. The orthoptist may perform nonsurgical treatments of patients with certain vision problems. An orthoptist frequently serves as a liaison between the ophthalmologist and the patient, explaining and carrying out some treatments.

FINDING OUT WHAT IS WRONG

Eye tests range from simple tests of vision involving reading the letters on an eye chart aloud to complicated hospital tests that are minor operations in themselves. This is because the conditions that they are designed to detect also vary considerably, from the measurement of near- or farsightedness—not strictly an eye health issue at all— to the investigation of medical conditions that could, if left untreated, result in blindness.

Eye tests

An optometrist can learn a surprising amount about your eye health as well as your vision from tests carried out in the consulting room. When necessary, a patient will be referred for further tests by an ophthalmologist and a specialist team.

WITH THE OPTOMETRIST

The primary role of the optometrist is to define and correct problems with the eye's focusing system. In addition, optometrists have a vital frontline role in the identification of potential eye health problems. They pick up signs of eye diseases such as glaucoma far more often than do family doctors. However, family doctors also have a major role in the detection of eye disease. An optometrist who suspects that there is a problem with eye health always refers the patient to a doctor, and eye conditions such as infections should prompt the sufferer to see a doctor, not an optometrist.

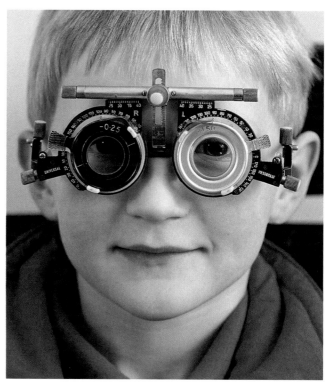

Trial frames
Trial frames, or test frames, hold sample lenses in place while the optometrist tests a patient's vision. The optometrist keeps changing the lenses until the correct strength of lens for each eye has been determined.

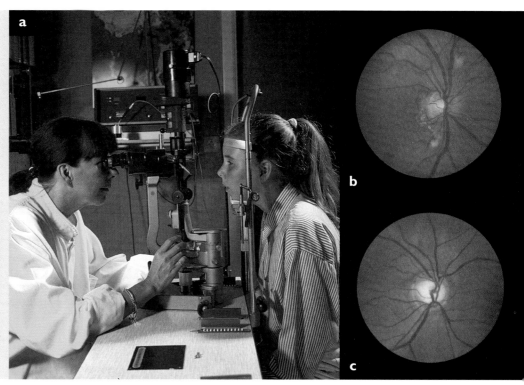

A slit lamp ophthalmoscope

a An eye doctor looks into the eyepiece of a slit lamp ophthalmoscope in order to see the back of the retina in the patient's eye. The instrument directs a fine beam of light into the eye and contains lenses that allow a magnified view of where the light falls.

b The retina of a healthy eye looks like this. Blood vessels radiate from the optic disk that marks the spot where the optic nerve leaves the eye; this causes the so-called blind spot.

c An ophthalmoscopic image of the retina of a patient with glaucoma reveals that the optic disk has a larger central pale area, or "cup."

AT THE EYE DOCTOR

An optometrist who suspects that a patient may have, for example, glaucoma, refers the patient to his or her family doctor. The doctor then makes a referral for the patient to be examined by an ophthalmologist. It is at this visit that further tests are done that enable the ophthalmologist to make a definite diagnosis. (Twice as many patients are sent for tests for suspected glaucoma as turn out to have the disease.) Optometrists don't have the time, equipment, or training to make definite diagnoses themselves.

MEASURING THE SIZE OF REFRACTION

Tests measuring problems such as nearsightedness (myopia) or farsightedness (hypermetropia), known as refractive errors, are carried out by an optometrist. If serious enough, a reduction in vision can usually be corrected by glasses or contact lenses.

To determine the size of refraction, the optometrist places lenses of different strengths in front of each eye until the lens that provides the best vision is identified. This is done by dropping the lenses into a specialized pair of glasses frames (a trial frame) or by using an instrument called a phoropter, which looks like a large pair of goggles and contains all necessary lenses.

While the test is carried out, the patient looks into the distance with focusing relaxed and then at the distance of close tasks, such as reading and sewing. This is particularly important for patients older than 45, because focusing ability reduces with age, so the prescription required for distance vision is different from that for near sight. Distance vision is commonly tested by asking the patient to read letters of a decreasing size from a chart placed 20 feet away. The test result is written as a prescription, which can be made into a pair of glasses or contact lenses (see page 100).

ORTHOPTIC TESTS

There are a number of simple but ingenious tests for investigating how well a patient's eyes are working together and how well they are able to focus. Different tests are carried out depending on the nature of the patient's symptoms (if any).

Simply by asking the patient to move his or her eyes in different directions or to focus at different distances, an optometrist is able to determine a remarkable amount about the patient's extraocular muscles (those that control eye movement) and focusing muscles. If necessary, glasses or contact lenses will be prescribed in order to correct problems or weaknesses detected.

SCANNING THE RETINA

Inside the back of the eye is the retina. The cells of the retina are connected to the brain via the optic nerve. Any problems with the retina or optic nerve can result in a potentially permanent reduction of vision, so an optometrist will always scan the back of the eye to ensure that it is healthy.

Scanning the back of the eye can be performed either with an instrument called an ophthalmoscope or by using a separate focusing lens and a light source (a slit lamp). The light and lenses of either instrument are focused on the patient's retina. The eye doctor or optometrist then looks at the optic nerve, the blood vessels, the retinal tissue, and the clear jellylike fluid in front of the retina. Sometimes eye drops are used to dilate the pupil or make it bigger temporarily; this enables the eye doctor to see more of the retina.

As well as diagnosing specific eye problems by viewing the retina, an eye doctor may detect general systemic illnesses. For example, diseases such as glaucoma and tumors can damage the optic nerve, and hypertension (high blood pressure) and diabetes can cause blood vessel changes, bleeding, and an accumulation of fluid. If detected early, a number of these changes can be treated before they cause permanent loss of vision.

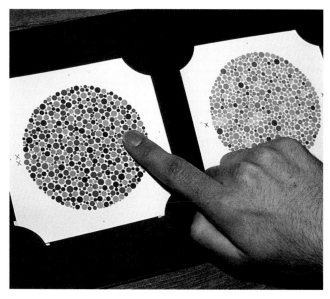

Standard color blindness tests
Color blindness is much more common in men than in women and in those of European descent than in Asians or Africans. Tests usually consist of "hidden" numbers or shapes in a colored pattern; a diagnosis is made on the basis of several different patterns.

VIEWING THE ANTERIOR EYE

The anterior eye is any part of the eye that is in front of the retina. This includes the lens, iris, cornea, sclera, conjunctiva, eyelid, and lashes, as well as the fluid within the eye. An optometrist checks for any abnormalities or diseases and can investigate problems such as cataracts, corneal scarring, eyelid lesions or pigmentation, and eye infections such as conjunctivitis and keratitis. The examination is usually performed using a slit lamp, which is essentially a magnifier with a light source.

COLOR BLINDNESS TESTS

Approximately 1 in 12 males and 1 in 200 females have abnormal color vision. In very rare cases, this may mean having no color vision—seeing only in shades of gray—but in most cases it involves varying amounts of difficulty distinguishing between certain colors, usually reds and greens. It is important for someone who has abnormal color vision to be aware of this at an early age, because a number of occupations, including firefighting, textile working, commercial piloting, and electrical work require normal color vision.

An optometrist can carry out a simple color vision test involving a series of plates or pages with colored numbers or dots. The patient has to identify the numbers or choose a colored dot that is different from others. These plates appear different according to the patient's disability. Further tests are available that more fully describe the type and severity of a defect and usually involve arranging colored pieces in order of tonal variation.

EYE PRESSURE MEASUREMENT (TONOMETRY)

Between the cornea and lens, the eye is filled with aqueous humor—a clear fluid that is constantly being produced and drained away. The presence of this fluid creates a pressure within the eye known as intraocular pressure (IOP). If the IOP is elevated, the pressure within the eye increases and can damage the optic nerve. Because abnormal pressure does not usually cause symptoms until it is very high, the pressure should be measured from time to time. Eye pressure tests are most often carried out as checks for indications of the common condition glaucoma, in which eyesight deteriorates because of elevated IOP. The tests used to measure the IOP work on the principle that the force required to flatten a given area of the cornea is proportional to the pressure inside the eye. There are two methods of performing this test:

Testing the visual field

Measuring a patient's visual field checks the extent to which she or he can see centrally and peripherally. Loss of vision can occur in the central vision, peripheral (side) vision, or both.

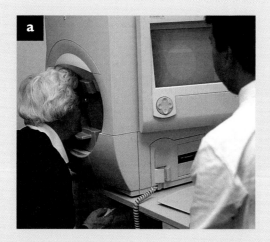

a An instrument known as a perimeter is used to map the extent of the patient's visual field. Seated in front of the perimeter, the patient observes a central fixating spot while small lights of variable brightness are flashed around the surrounding bowl-like or flat area. The patient indicates whether or not he or she can see the lights, and from these responses, a printout can be made of the extent of the patient's field of vision.

b Loss of visual field can be caused by damage to the visual pathway, including the retina, the optic nerve (as with glaucoma), and parts of the brain. Different problems give rise to different patterns of visual field loss as detected by the perimeter.

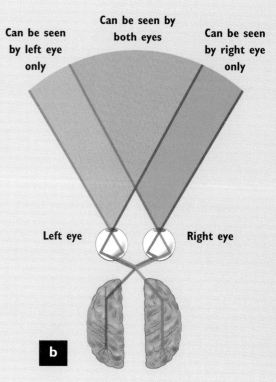

- **Applanation tonometry** A flat-ended probe is placed onto the eye after the instillation of anesthetic eye drops.
- **Noncontact tonometry** A short, sharp puff of air is blown into the eye, resulting in the flattening of the cornea. This is normally done three times in succession for each eyeball. This standard test for glaucoma should be performed as part of every eye checkup for anyone who is over 40 or has a family history of glaucoma.

IMAGING THE EYES

Sometimes it is necessary to obtain images of a patient's eyes. Eye doctors have used cameras for a number of years to image both the front of the eye and the retina. Digital cameras linked to computer programs that enable the storage, analysis, editing, and e-mailing of images, as required, are now used.

In terms of retinal imaging, technology is improving all the time. A scanning laser ophthalmoscope uses laser technology to provide highly magnified images of the retina. It is able to show very early changes in retinal structure and can also provide three-dimensional images.

FLUORESCEIN ANGIOGRAPHY

Fluorescein angiography is a technique carried out at the eye clinic to investigate the retinal blood vessels. A fluorescent dye is injected into a patient's bloodstream, and after a short time, it reaches the blood vessels in the eye. The vessels then show up on images taken of the retina. Leakages of blood vessels show up as bright areas, and areas of the retina that are not receiving sufficient blood will appear dark. This technique is often used to investigate sources of bleeding in conditions such as diabetic retinopathy and age-related macular degeneration.

Testing for diabetic retinopathy
Fluorescein angiogram of the retina of the eye of a person with diabetic retinopathy. This occurs when diabetes damages the blood vessels of the retina. These damaged vessels can leak or become blocked.

CURRENT TREATMENTS

Treatments for eyes fall into two categories. Most common are treatments for problems with focusing. Usually, the solution is to wear glasses or contact lenses to correct the fault. Only in recent years has surgery begun to be used to reduce near- or farsightedness by altering the lens within the eye. Then there are treatments for problems of eye health. Sore, inflamed, or dry eyes from infections and allergies are treated with eye drops or ointment. Surgical removal is the cure for cataracts, and surgery is often the best treatment for retinal detachment and tumors. The precision and effectiveness of eye surgery have been revolutionized by the introduction of lasers, ultrasound, the operating microscope, and microinstruments.

Corrective lenses

The range of glasses and contact lenses available to those who are near- or farsighted is greater than ever, and it addresses fashion considerations as well as those of vision. There are also various options for people with a combination of requirements.

UNDERSTANDING A PRESCRIPTION

- **Nearsightedness** A prescription for this is preceded by a minus sign, such as R: –3.00, L: –3.50. These "minus lenses" have a concave surface, which causes light rays to diverge a little before entering the eye.
- **Farsightedness** A prescription for this is preceded by a plus sign, such as R: +1.50, L: +1.25, and these lenses are sometimes called "plus lenses." They have a convex surface, which causes light rays to converge a little before entering the eye.
- **Astigmatism** If a patient has astigmatism, the lenses prescribed will have a cylindrical shape built into them. The prescription includes an extra number to define the power and position of the cylinder—for example R: –2.00/–1.75 x 115. These lenses correct the difference in the light-bending properties of different parts of the cornea.

GLASSES

Glasses remain the most popular choice for correcting vision. An individual may need lenses of different powers to see clearly at different distances, but this does not necessarily mean needing more than one pair of glasses.

Single vision or multifocal?

Spectacle lenses are made in two basic forms. Single-vision lenses provide correction for a single prescription. Multifocal lenses enable more than one prescription to be built into the lens, and one pair of glasses could suit a range of different activities. However, it takes longer for some wearers to get used to them than others.

- **Bifocals** have two prescriptions, a top one for distance and a bottom one for near vision. The size and shape of the two areas can vary to suit individual needs, and sometimes there is a visible dividing line between them.
- **Trifocal lenses** include three corrections for three different working distances—distance at the top, mid-distance in the center, and near at the bottom.

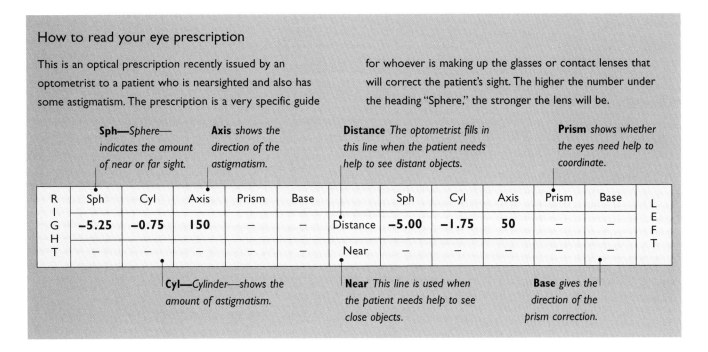

How to read your eye prescription

This is an optical prescription recently issued by an optometrist to a patient who is nearsighted and also has some astigmatism. The prescription is a very specific guide for whoever is making up the glasses or contact lenses that will correct the patient's sight. The higher the number under the heading "Sphere," the stronger the lens will be.

Sph—Sphere— *indicates the amount of near or far sight.*

Axis *shows the direction of the astigmatism.*

Distance *The optometrist fills in this line when the patient needs help to see distant objects.*

Prism *shows whether the eyes need help to coordinate.*

RIGHT	Sph	Cyl	Axis	Prism	Base		Sph	Cyl	Axis	Prism	Base	LEFT
	−5.25	−0.75	150	−	−	Distance	−5.00	−1.75	50	−	−	
	−	−	−	−	−	Near	−	−	−	−	−	

Cyl—Cylinder—*shows the amount of astigmatism.*

Near *This line is used when the patient needs help to see close objects.*

Base *gives the direction of the prism correction.*

- **Varifocal or progressive lenses** are like trifocals but have the advantage of no visible lines, so they look just like single-vision lenses.
- **Single-vision lenses** for someone who only needs help with close work can be mounted in "half-eye" frames that enable the wearer to look through the lenses when reading and above the lenses to see into the distance.

Glass or plastic?

There are three main types of lens material: plastic, glass, and polycarbonate (a form of hard plastic). Each has its advantages and disadvantages. Plastic is light but easily scratched. Glass is less easily scratched but heavier and more dangerous if broken. Polycarbonate is impact resistant, making it a good choice for children, athletes, and workers who need eye protection; it is light, but lenses are easily scratched and can give distorted vision to wearers with high prescriptions.

Thinner lenses

Glass and plastic lenses can be made with "higher refractive indexes" that allow the lenses to be thinner than they would be otherwise, improving the cosmetic appearance of lenses made to high prescriptions. (The refractive index of a lens is a measure of how much the lens bends the rays of light that pass through it.)

Coatings and tints

Plastic lenses generally have an antiscratch coating. An antireflection coating on glass or plastic helps protect the eyes from glare and also makes lenses look thinner and less noticeable. Tints in lenses are used for sun or glare protection or are worn simply as a fashion accessory. Gray tints are the best choice for car drivers because they will not distort color perception. Photochromic lenses contain special dyes that darken when exposed to sunlight and lighten when protection is not required.

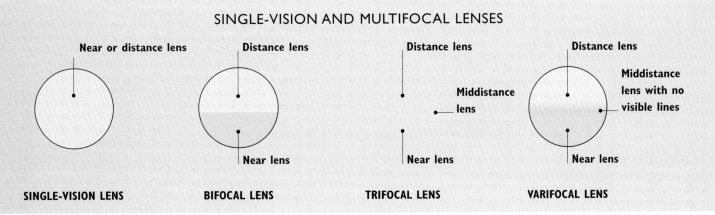

SINGLE-VISION AND MULTIFOCAL LENSES

Near or distance lens

Distance lens

Near lens

Distance lens

Middistance lens

Near lens

Distance lens

Middistance lens with no visible lines

Near lens

SINGLE-VISION LENS **BIFOCAL LENS** **TRIFOCAL LENS** **VARIFOCAL LENS**

CONTACT LENSES

Tremendous advances have been made in contact lens technology in recent years. The effort needed to take care of contact lenses is less than before—and there are even types of lenses that require no cleaning at all. There are now very few people for whom contact lenses are not suitable. Because contact lenses are worn directly on the eye, wearers enjoy greater all-around vision than with glasses and the lenses do not fog up in wet weather. The plastic lens allows oxygen to pass through to the eye, which helps keep the eye healthy.

Correction of near- and farsightedness follows the same principles as for glasses, and there are single-vision and multifocal contact lenses. Tinted contact lenses can change eye color, but because there is no color in the central part of the lens, they don't tint the wearer's vision.

- **Soft lenses** made of soft plastic are worn by four out of five contact lens wearers. There are "continuous wear" and "daily disposable" soft lenses; there are also special lenses for those who need extra oxygen flow to the eye surface, have dry or sensitive eyes, or work in smoky atmospheres.
- **Gas-permeable lenses** are made from a semirigid plastic and therefore take a little longer to get used to than soft lenses.

Contact lenses and astigmatism

Mild astigmatism can be corrected by an ordinary gas-permeable lens because its semirigid, spherical shape overlies the football-shaped cornea. For those with higher levels of astigmatism or who prefer a soft lens, a special design called a toric lens has a cylinder built into the lens and is available in gas-permeable and soft lenses.

Contact lenses and presbyopia

There are various options for contact lens wearers when they become presbyopic in early middle age.

- Varifocal contact lenses work similarly to glasses lenses in that two prescriptions are built into each lens.
- People who are nearsighted can wear contact lenses for distance vision and glasses on top for reading.
- An alternative is to wear a contact lens in one eye for distance vision and a lens in the other eye for near vision. After a few days, the brain adjusts to this and the wearer experiences clear vision at both distances.

The risk of infection

Because contact lenses are worn against the eye, careless lens handling invites infection. Contact lens wearers should always wash their hands before touching lenses or eyes and follow lens care instructions to the letter.

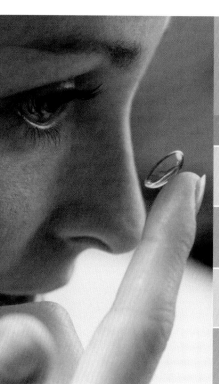

What types of contact lenses are available?

A decade ago, most contact lens wearers had one pair of lenses, which they took out and cleaned every night. This is still the most common way of wearing and caring for gas-permeable lenses. However, for soft lenses, there are now daily disposable lenses and also continuous wear lenses that are worn all the time, for up to a month.

Type	Description	Advantages	Additional information
SOFT	Made of a soft, flexible plastic that drapes over the eye.	Easier to adapt to at first use and more comfortable overall than semirigid lenses.	They are more easily damaged than semirigid lenses and are generally less long-lasting.
GAS-PERMEABLE	Made from semirigid plastic; smaller than soft lenses.	More suitable for those with astigmatism than most soft lenses.	Take longer to get used to than soft lenses; may be harder to insert and remove.
CONTINUOUS WEAR	Soft lenses worn 24 hours a day for as long as a month.	No need to take out and clean lenses at the end of each day.	Today there is less chance of eye infection from these lenses than in the past.
DAILY DISPOSABLE	Soft lenses that are removed and discarded every night.	No need to clean lenses at the end of each day.	These are generally more expensive than soft lenses if you wear them every day.

Drug treatments for eyes

Eye drops and ointments are most commonly used to treat infection and inflammation of the eye. Drops are also a suitable way of administering the drugs needed to treat glaucoma, to soothe allergic reactions, and to treat the irritating condition known as dry eye.

ANTIBIOTICS FOR CONJUNCTIVITIS

A bacterial infection can be treated with an antibacterial preparation applied to the eye as drops or ointment or sometimes both. Eye ointment is usually applied at night and eye drops during the day. The active ingredient is often an antibiotic, commonly chloramphenicol. With chloramphenicol, two drops are instilled into the affected eye at least every 2 hours for the first 24 hours and reduced to four times daily as the infection is controlled. The drops are continued for 48 hours after the infection has cleared. Other antibiotics that may be used are gentamicin, neomycin, and fusidic acid. Newer antibacterial eye drops with a wider spectrum of activity include ciprofloxacin and ofloxacin.

EYE DROPS FOR GLAUCOMA

Treatment aims to reduce pressure within the eye (the intraocular pressure) by lessening the production of aqueous humor or increasing its outflow. In this way, further deterioration of the field of vision is prevented.
- **Beta-blockers** are the first-choice drugs for lowering eye pressure in the U.S. A beta-blocker such as timolol treats mild glaucoma by reducing the rate of production of aqueous humor. A beta-blocker should not be given to patients with asthma or those with obstructive airway disease or heart problems.
- **Prostaglandins** are the second-choice eye drop if beta-blockers are no longer effective or if it becomes unwise to take them for some other reason. The market leader, latanoprost, is at least as effective as the best beta-blockers. Prostaglandins have not replaced beta-blockers

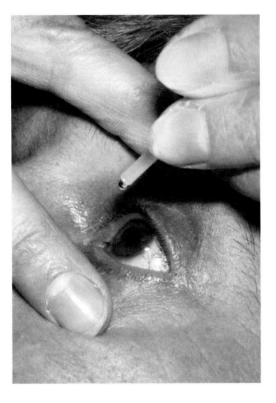

A drop in the eye
Eye drops deliver the drug treatment of choice directly to the surface of the eye, ensuring maximum impact.

in the U.S., however, because they all—and latanoprost in particular—stimulate melanin production in the iris and thus can turn light eyes brown. They also stimulate eyelash growth.
- **Brimonidine** is used quite frequently with a beta-blocker or alone.

DROPS FOR ALLERGIES

Eye drops containing corticosteroids or other anti-inflammatory preparations are used to treat allergic eye conditions (see page 68). Prednisolone steroid eye drops, nedocrimil, and lodoxamide are the main medications. Sodium cromoglycate is also popular. Emedastine and levocabastine are also used.

OVER-THE-COUNTER EYE DROPS
- **For minor infections of the eyes and eyelids** Their main ingredient is propamidine, which is antibacterial, and they are to be used for 2 days, after which you should see a doctor if there is no improvement.
- **For minor eye irritations** Causes for this include smoky or dusty surroundings, driving, or close work. These drops usually have witch hazel as their main ingredient.
- **Artificial tear fluid** These treat the symptoms of dry eyes (see page 138) by covering the eye surface with a moist film that substitutes for the tear fluid that normally protects and lubricates the eye. Although artificial tears are designed to be nonirritating, an adverse reaction is possible, so contact lens wearers should consult their optometrist before using these drops.

Surgical treatments for eyes

New microsurgical techniques and computer-controlled lasers have made eye surgery an incredibly precise and accurate process, enabling reduced healing times and dramatic results unheard of just a few years ago.

A SIMPLE RETINAL DETACHMENT

The vitreous humor—the jellylike material that fills the body of the eye—is in contact with the retina and part of the role of the vitreous is to cushion it. With aging or as the result of injury, the vitreous may partly detach from the retina, causing a posterior vitreous detachment (a PVD). Pulling of the partly detached vitreous can tear the retina; fluid is then able to seep through these breaks in the retina and separate the retina from the retinal pigment epithelium. People who are very nearsighted are particularly prone to PVD and its consequences.

Early signs of a problem

We all sometimes see black dots, called floaters, but PVD is associated with the release of showers of floaters, and the retinal disturbance produces what appears to be flashing lights. In the early stages, however, the patient may not notice any deterioration in vision, and therefore these signs are often disregarded until the condition has become more advanced and there is some level of visual loss that prompts the patient to arrange an eye checkup.

Treatment options for a simple detachment

If retinal holes and tears are identified before detachment begins, then treatment may be a simple outpatient procedure, with the eye doctor using either an argon laser or a cryoprobe to seal all the breaks in the retina. If a detachment has taken place, surgery is the answer. The surgeon aims to relieve the pulling produced by the partly attached vitreous, close all of the retinal holes, and allow the retina to return to normal. Depending on the complexity of the detachment, the surgeon will opt for either scleral buckling or vitrectomy.

Scleral buckling surgery

The surgeon indents the wall of the eye close to the detachment so that by distorting the eye in this way, there is no longer a detachment. Retinal tears and holes are sealed externally with a cryoprobe, and subretinal fluid may be removed by a narrow-gauge needle. Thereafter, a silicone band (called an explant) is secured in place with sutures to maintain the indentation. Sometimes it is necessary to introduce a bubble of gas mixture or silicone oil into the vitreous cavity to help close retinal breaks.

Vitrectomy

A vitrectomy is performed if the vitreous pulling on the retina is particularly troublesome and it is thought necessary to remove the bulk of it and also if retinal holes and tears are large, dispersed, or hard to locate. The surgeon uses a special probe that both cuts and sucks up the vitreous. A fine fiberoptic light tube is also introduced into the vitreal cavity so that the surgeon can see clearly enough to treat all retinal holes, tears and breaks. Saline

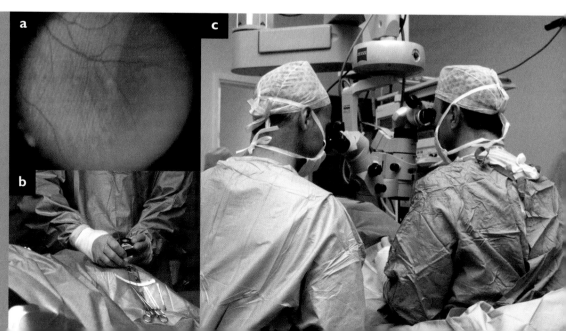

Retinal detachment repair by vitrectomy

a The detached part of the retina is the less brightly colored area to the right on this image.

b The eye has been immobilized and the pupil dilated for examination.

c During the operation, the surgeon and assistant use a ceiling-mounted microscope to see as clearly as possible.

ON THE CUTTING EDGE

Macular relocation surgery

Macular relocation surgery is a new treatment for patients who have recently lost vision from the wet form of age-related macular degeneration (AMD), in which a rapid development of vascular scar tissue near or under the macula (the part of the retina with the greatest concentration of light-sensitive cones) has reduced central vision. Sometimes a surgeon can detach the retina and macula and then reposition the macula on healthy tissue away from the vascular scarring so that it has a chance to survive and function well once again. This operation is still being refined; it can be very successful, but there have been frequent failures. When fully perfected, the operation will help some AMD sufferers, but unfortunately it is not a solution for the vast majority of AMD patients.

solution is introduced into the eye to replace vitreous that has been removed, and it is normal to introduce gas or silicone oil bubbles to help plug holes and reestablish retinal contact with the pigment epithelium.

Posturing after surgery

Patients with oil or gas bubbles in their vitreous may be required to "posture" during the recovery period after surgery. This may involve lying face down on a bed or leaning forward while sitting in a chair so that the bubble is in the best position possible for establishing reattachment of the retina. The patient may have to maintain this position—as much as possible—for a few days. A gas bubble disappears over time; silicone oil does not, so some surgeons like to remove it once reattachment is well established.

COMPLEX RETINAL DETACHMENTS

Fewer than 1 in 10 retinal detachments require further surgery. When this is necessary, it is generally because scar tissue has formed within the eye on the surface of the retina. Scar tissue on the retina prevents retinal reattachment, and when it contracts, it peels even more of the retina away from the retinal pigment epithelium, causing a tractional detachment.

Surgical solutions

The surgeon peels the scar tissue away from the retinal surface and chops it up with a vitrectomy cutter. In this way, the tension on the retina is relieved, allowing it to go back into place. Usually there are many more holes, breaks, and tears to deal with than is the case with a simple detachment. A gas mixture or silicone oil is needed within the vitreal cavity to promote the healing and adhesion process. Surgery of this type is on the cutting edge of ocular microsurgical development.

CORNEAL GRAFTS

Damage to the cornea caused by injury, infection, or disease can result in the cornea becoming cloudy and causing the patient's sight to deteriorate. If the cloudiness persists despite nonsurgical treatment and vision is not improved by glasses or contact lenses, then a corneal graft may be the answer.

The operation

The cloudy cornea is removed and replaced by a round segment of clear cornea from a donor, which, having been cut to a button shape by a sharp punchlike instrument called a trephine, is stitched into place on the recipient's eye. The transplant is usually a total replacement of the patient's cornea, but sometimes, if the problem is localized close to the corneal surface, a partial-thickness procedure is used by the surgeon. It sounds simple, but this delicate operation can take 1 to 2 hours.

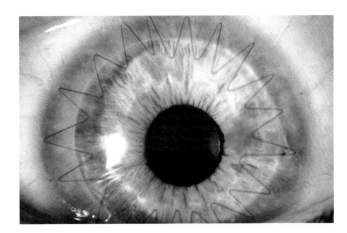

A patient's eye after a total corneal transplant
The stitching can be clearly seen surrounding the grafted cornea. The suture thread used for this operation is remarkably fine, but even so, the healing in the cornea is slow and the stitches may need to be in place for as long as 2 years.

After the operation

With the transplant protected by a pad and cover, the patient is fit to go home after a couple of days. The healing process is slow, so strenuous activities must be avoided for several months. Corneal grafting has a better than 80 percent chance of success. Because the cornea does not have blood vessels, lymphocytes and other cells that cause rejection of "foreign tissue" do not usually cause a problem. It is not necessary to tissue-type donor and host before uncomplicated corneal grafting procedures (a process that is essential if kidney and liver transplants are to have any chance of success).

Unfortunately, some patients, particularly those with a disorder in which there has been blood vessel invasion of the corneal tissue, do reject corneal transplants. In such cases, patient-donor blood matching is carried out and long-term topical steroid medication may be needed to moderate any reaction to the graft.

Donation and storage

Tissue for corneal grafting can be stored in a laboratory for a few days without increasing the risk of graft failure. There is some risk of a corneal transplant passing virus infections such as AIDS and hepatitis to the host, so every donor is screened before the corneas are used. Fewer people are willing to donate their eyes in the event of their death than are willing to give their heart, liver, or kidneys, so finding a donor can be a problem.

SIGHT CORRECTION BY SURGERY

Alternatives to sight correction by glasses or contact lenses are procedures known as photorefractive surgery. The aim is to alter the corneal curvature sufficiently to provide, as closely as possible, the appropriate refractive correction. Surgery is generally used to combat nearsightedness; farsightedness can also be corrected but less straightforwardly, and therefore operations to correct farsightedness are not as frequently performed.

Radial keratotomy (RK)

RK was first developed in the former Soviet Union in the late 1970s and early 1980s. This procedure treats nearsightedness by using a scalpel to make a series of radial cuts around the edges of the cornea to flatten the corneal curvature. The more nearsighted the individual, the more incisions are necessary. Because of this, this treatment is best suited to those who are not very

Correcting a squint by surgery

a This boy has a convergent squint, with the left eye turning in toward the nose.
b First, the surgeon must weaken the medial rectal muscle on the inner side of the eye, which is turning the eye too far inward. To do this, the surgeon begins by snipping the muscle free from the eyeball.
c Then the surgeon measures a few millimeters back from the muscle's original point of attachment and stitches the free end of the muscle in place in this new position.
d Now the surgeon needs to strengthen the lateral rectus muscle (on the outer side of the eye) so that it will do a better job of pulling the eye outward.
e The lateral rectus muscle is cut, shortened, and then stitched back in place in its original position on the eyeball.
f The operation has been a success—the patient's eyes are now in alignment. The redness in the left eye will clear up in a matter of weeks as the eye recovers from the operation.

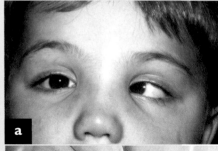
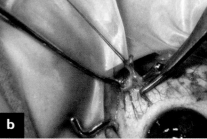
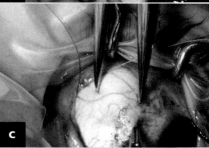
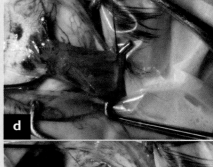
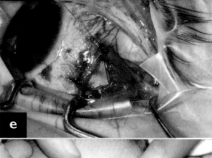
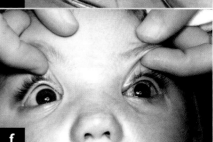

HAVING LASER SURGERY (LASIK) TO CORRECT NEARSIGHTEDNESS

After years of monitoring the progress of laser eye surgery for nearsightedness and astigmatism, I finally felt that the procedure was commonplace enough for me to seriously look into it..

I prepared for my initial consultation by not wearing my gas-permeable lenses for several weeks, allowing my eyes to fully return to their natural shape. At the consultation, my nearsightedness and astigmatism were measured, as was the thickness of both corneas. I knew there was a chance my eyes wouldn't be suitable, but I was told that a successful outcome was very likely. The operation—using a technique known as LASIK—took place a few days later. First, I received anesthetic eye drops and then I was directed to a

chair that reclined so my head was lower than my feet. A spreader kept my left eyelid open, the lashes were taped down, and my chair was swayed beneath the laser. A suction ring was put on my eyeball to keep it still.

Next, with a noise like a pneumatic drill, a laser cut a flap through the top of my cornea. The flap was folded back and the cornea beneath was then reshaped by the laser. While this was going on I smelt something burning—it was the smell of the tissue evaporating. The reshaping complete, the flap was folded back in place; the suction ring, spreader and tape were removed; and a clear plastic shield was taped over my eye. The surgeon assured me that the flap would quickly bond in place.

Then my right eye was treated. I had felt no pain at all in my left eye, but I felt discomfort—even pain—in my right eye. It was a relief when the procedure ended.

Twenty minutes later, I left for home; I could take the shields off at home but had to wear them for the first 3 nights. The next day, I was told my left eye had almost perfect vision and my right eye was nearly as good. My eyesight fluctuated (as expected) for 5 or 6 weeks before settling. There was some bruising and for a while I experienced severe glare around lights and road signs when driving after dark. At my final checkup, 2 months after the operation, it was confirmed that I no longer needed contact lenses.

nearsighted. RK has now largely been superseded by laser surgery, in part because it has been found that scalpel cuts tend to weaken the eye.

Photorefractive keratectomy (PRK)

PRK has been in use for about 10 years now. The technique relies on the remarkable properties of the excimer laser. This laser is the perfect microscalpel and produces a microscopic vaporisation of tissue with each pulse without any adjacent damage. The excimer, under computer control, can be used for sculpting out segments of the cornea very precisely and accurately.

In the PRK procedure, the surface epithelium is removed after the administration of anesthetic drops. The computer then sculpts the underlying tissue to produce the required alteration in corneal curvature. Most patients treated are nearsighted, but the program can be adjusted to treat farsighted individuals and those with corneal astigmatism.

PRK is not problem-free, however. The sculpting is done in the surface layers of the cornea, where sensory nerve endings are abundant, which means that there is

some pain in the first week after surgery while the epithelium is healing. Healing is slow; it may take up to 6 months to reach best vision. In the short term, some patients experience haze, glare, and halos. Infection is not common, but it can occur. Some loss of correction is a long-term disappointment most frequently experienced by those who are particularly nearsighted or astigmatic.

Laser-assisted in-situ keratomileusis (LASIK)

LASIK is a new procedure, popular in the United States. LASIK overcomes some of the side effects of PRK because the surgeon cuts a flap in the cornea and then performs the excimer laser procedure in the deeper regions of the cornea, where there are fewer nerve endings. As a result, LASIK patients are more comfortable in the immediate postoperative period than their PRK counterparts and, in addition, the healing period appears to be shorter than after PRK. There is no significant difference in visual outcome between the two techniques. It looks as if LASIK is likely to replace PRK, but the long-term outcome for patients who have undergone the LASIK procedure is as yet unknown.

Removing a cataract

A cataract occurs when the lens within the eye becomes cloudy, reducing the amount of light reaching the retina. Cataract surgery is safe and quick. The lens of the eye is removed and replaced with an artificial one made of plastic.

A cataract can show up in childhood, it can develop after an injury to the eye, or it can be associated with systemic diseases such as diabetes, but by far the most common cause is old age. There is no medical cure and no prospect of one as yet, but surgery to remove and replace the cataractous lens is one of the most successful operations available today, and 80 to 90 percent of patients attain 6/12 vision or better (the level needed to be able to drive a car).

Over the past 20 years, there have been radical changes in the way eye surgeons treat cataracts. The new keyhole surgery techniques are minimally invasive, so surgery is much less traumatic than in the past. Patients who are otherwise healthy can be home the same day, with the whole operation usually done as an outpatient procedure under local anesthetic.

The other major breakthrough has been the development of plastic lenses to replace the "natural" lens. A plastic intraocular lens is fitted into the capsular bag in the last stage of cataract surgery. The use of intraocular plastic lenses has largely done away with the need for the "cataract glasses," which had very powerful convex lenses that were needed when the eye did not have its own lens. Plastic intraocular lenses have been in routine use since the 1970s.

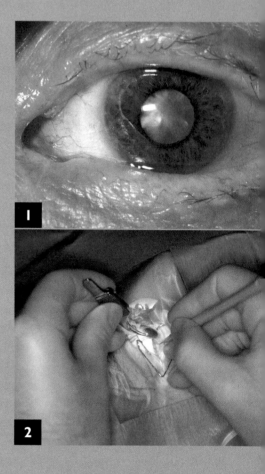

1

2

Training for cataract surgery

Cataract operations are relatively quick and have a high success rate, but that doesn't make them easy to perform. The training of cataract surgeons takes several years. In the U.S., in particular, eye surgeons train with the help of virtual reality simulations, using computer-generated imagery to practice before operating on real patients. Because of the lengthy and costly training, there are far too few cataract surgeons in third-world countries. As a result, cataracts are still the biggest cause of blindness worldwide; 15 million cataract blind is a conservative estimate of the numbers.

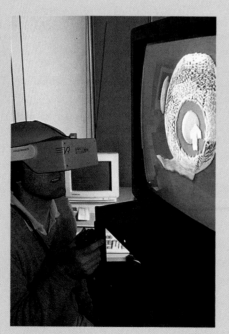

The procedure step by step

1 A typical cataract—an opaque lens—that requires surgical removal. Preparation for cataract removal begins with the patient being given eye drops to enlarge the pupil as much as possible. A fully dilated pupil will give the surgeon better access to the cataract that lies behind it. Local anesthetic is given by means of an injection that immobilizes the muscles attached to the eye and numbs the eye and surrounding area.

2 The surgeon makes a small incision through the cornea to gain access to the lens beneath it. The lens lies within a tough, transparent membranous capsule.

3 Throughout the operation, the surgeon views the eye through an operating microscope that greatly enlarges the image of the operation site. The surgeon's view can be seen on the

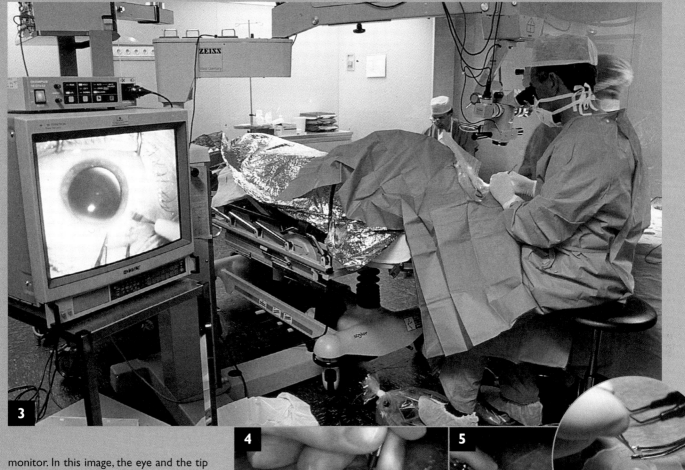

3

monitor. In this image, the eye and the tip of a high-frequency ultrasound probe are clearly visible.

4 The surgeon inserts the probe into the lens capsule, where ultrasound breaks up the lens material that lies within the lens capsule. The lens matter is then sucked up through a fine tube within the probe. This process is known as phacoemulsification.

5 A replacement lens is slipped into the lens capsule that still remains in the eye. Inset: A prosthetic crystalline eye lens is held by forceps before insertion into the eye. The new lens is folded and pushed through the incision into the lens capsule, then unfolded and positioned correctly within the capsule.

6 Very fine stitches are used to close the opening in the eye needed to introduce the new lens. Then an eye pad is placed over the eye and the operation is over.

4

5

The patient can generally go home on the same day. Eye drops containing antibiotics and steroids help keep infection and inflammation at bay. The sutures are removed at a later date, again as an outpatient procedure, under local anesthetic in drop form. The new lens generally gives excellent distance vision, but glasses are usually necessary for close vision.

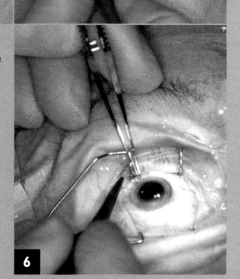

6

Ocular tumors

Although it's possible for a whole range of tumors—both benign and malignant—to develop in the eyelids and soft tissues that surround the eye, cancers with tumors that are actually inside the eye itself fortunately are very rare.

Cancer of the eye most commonly occurs when secondary tumor cells seeded from tumors of the breast, lungs, or intestines, for example, lodge in the eye. Of cancers that occur in the eye as their primary location, there are two of significance: retinoblastoma and ocular melanoma. The first is associated with children, the second with adults.

RETINOBLASTOMA

This tumor is very rare; it occurs in just 1 in every 18,000 babies. It is generally identified when children are between 1 and 3 years old; by 7 years of age, the risk of getting this cancer is past. It may occur in just one eye but can develop in both. Despite being so rare, it is well-known by doctors and scientists, and routine examinations check for it in the early years.

The tumor is inherited but can also develop spontaneously in children with no obvious family association. If there is a family history of retinoblastoma,

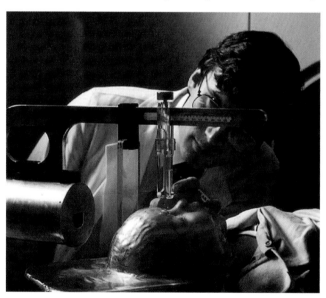

Radiotherapy for retinoblastoma
Before electron beam radiation for retinoblastoma, it is vital that the patient's retina be in precise alignment with the path of the electron beam (to avoid unnecessary damage to the eye). This is achieved by fixing the head in position with a plastic custom-made mask and then testing the alignment with a harmless red laser light, as shown above.

there is a 50 percent chance of a brother or sister developing the cancer; if there is no family history, the risk of a sibling developing retinoblastoma falls to less than 1 in 20.

A retinoblastoma results from the loss of function of a gene on chromosome 13, which normally produces a tumor suppression substance called RB protein. This protein prevents the uncontrolled growth of embryonic cells that, among other things, give rise to the rods and cones in the retina of the eye. Without RB protein or enough of it, a retinoblastoma can develop in the retina. If left untreated, the cancer will spread from the eye, with potentially fatal consequences.

How is the tumor treated?

Traditionally, treatment involved complete removal of the eye. Enucleation, as it is called, still has to be carried out if the tumor is particularly large, but this is not always the case. Retinoblastomas are sensitive to radiation, so preferred options include treatment with a radioactive plaque or a proton beam. Laser or cryotherapy (freezing the tumor) may get rid of the tumor if it is particularly small. If the tumor is small and away from the macula, the patient should retain reasonable to good sight; the larger and more central the retinoblastoma, the poorer the visual outcome.

OCULAR MELANOMA

Skin melanomas are on the rise and are rightly receiving considerable publicity, but many people are unaware that melanomas can also develop in the eye. The frequency of skin melanoma is closely linked to exposure to ultraviolet radiation from the sun, but the association between ocular melanoma and sunlight is less clear.

Ocular melanoma (see page 142), like skin melanoma, is a tumor that develops from pigmented cells called melanocytes. There are three sites within the eye where a melanoma can form: the choroid, the ciliary body that surrounds the iris, and the iris itself. Iris melanomas are the least common (8 percent of ocular melanomas), and choroidal melanomas are the most common (80 percent).

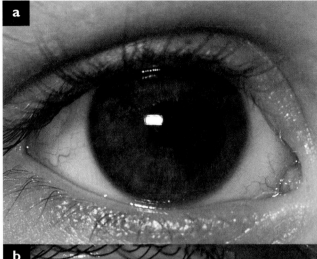

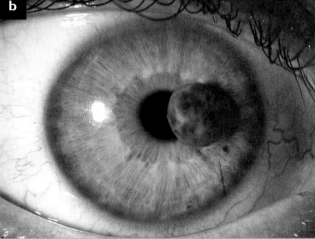

Iris melanomas—benign and malignant

a Not all iris melanomas are malignant. Shown here is a benign, harmless melanoma (nevus) within the eye of a 1-year-old boy. No treatment is needed.

b A malignant melanoma (as here) must be removed before it spreads to another part of the body. Not every iris melanoma is brown.

Adults over 65 years old are 10 times more likely to develop a choroidal melanoma than those under age 45. The choroid is the layer of the eye that lies immediately behind the retina. When a melanoma develops in the choroid, the melanoma pushes the retina forward, causing the retina to detach. Common symptoms are blurred vision, visual field loss, and a mass of "floaters." (These are the symptoms of all retinal detachments—only a very few of the many detachments seen at an eye clinic are the result of a malignancy.)

Ocular melanomas are rare among Africans and Asians. Blue-eyed people are at three times the risk of ocular melanoma than people with brown eyes.

How is the tumor treated?

Choroidal and ciliary body melanomas are both malignancies that seed tumor cells to distant organs—particularly the liver—and can have long-term fatal consequences. In the past, it was common to enucleate (remove) any eye diagnosed with ocular melanoma. Today, however, surgeons are far more conservative, and attempts are made to eliminate the cancer while leaving as much useful sight as possible. The eye is only removed if the melanoma is too large for effective treatment by some other means and the risk of the tumor spreading is too great.

There are various treatments available.

• **Small tumors**, particularly iris melanomas, may not require aggressive therapy and may even be safe enough to leave if there are no signs of growth.

• **Transpupillary thermotherapy (TTT)** treats small choroidal melanomas. This treatment uses an infrared laser to destroy the melanoma and is favored because it spares vision particularly well.

• **Plaque radiiation** is usually the first choice for small and medium-sized tumors. A radioactive plaque is placed over the site of the tumor for a number of days.

• **Proton-beam irradiation** is used effectively for larger and less accessible melanomas.

• **Surgery** does not have to involve removal of the whole eye. In some cases, the tumor can be removed, leaving the rest of the eye intact.

Artificial eyes

People who lose an eye, generally either through treatment for cancer or as the result of an accident, will be offered an artificial eye. These have improved enormously in appearance in recent years but are still less than perfect. They are made of plastic and consist of a shell fitted into the socket together with a front ocular prosthesis that can move.

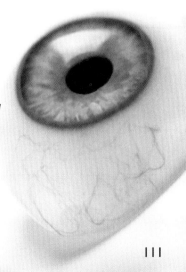

Knowing what can go wrong with the mouth

Dental disorders range from the very common to the extremely rare. For more common problems, knowing what can go wrong can play an important part in the prevention of disease. Early diagnosis of less-common disorders may help minimize dental problems in later life.

The most common disorders of the mouth are not only those that affect the teeth themselves (dental decay and tooth wear), but also those that affect the supporting tissues of the teeth—primarily the gums. The majority of the population of a Westernized society will suffer from at least one, if not all, of these conditions at some time. There are also thousands of other disorders that can affect the mouth, and these can be classified as developmental, traumatic, infectious, or neoplastic (that is, a tumor). In addition to taking care of the teeth and gums, avoiding heavy drinking and smoking will dramatically reduce the risk of oral problems.

Dental caries initially affects the enamel on the surface of the tooth, but with time it will spread to deeper layers and destroy the underlying dentin. If caries is left untreated, the bacteria in a progressing lesion will spread through the dentin into the pulp of the tooth, which contains the nerves that respond to pain. The pulp becomes inflamed, causing the symptoms of toothache, particularly localized pain and headaches, to appear.

Genetics play a part in dental caries; there is evidence that inherited disorders of tooth development that result in an altered structure of the enamel increase the risk of tooth decay.

MORE COMMON

ORAL HERPES	GUM DISEASE	TOOTH DECAY	CLEFT LIP AND/OR PALATE
Oral herpes, manifested as cold sores on the mouth, may affect as much as 50 to 80 percent of the adult population.	An estimated 80 percent of Americans have some form of periodontal disease	This is the most common chronic disease among children ages 5 to 17, with 59 percent suffering from it. Many adults—27 percent of those ages 35 to 44 and 30 percent of those 65 and older—also have untreated dental caries.	Cleft lip or cleft lip and palate occurs in 1 in 1000 babies. Cleft palate alone occurs in 1 in 2000 babies. Boys are affected more often.

DENTAL DECAY

Dental decay, or dental caries, remains the biggest problem for dentists to treat in both children and adults. It is a complex disorder that is driven by the ability of certain bacterial species—streptococci and lactobacilli—to metabolize sugars to acids, which then dissolve the structure of the tooth. The bacteria are not the only important factors to consider when evaluating an individual's susceptibility to dental caries, however. Diet is a major contributing factor, in particular the amount of sugar—both "natural" and refined—in the diet and the frequency with which sugary foods or drinks are consumed. The resistance of the teeth to caries is another significant factor. The major protecting factor is fluoride, which is administered most effectively through drinking water and fluoride toothpaste. Fluoride is naturally present in water in some parts of the country.

TOOTH WEAR

Tooth wear tends to be regarded as a more "contemporary" problem, and it is likely to become more prevalent as more people keep their natural teeth into old age. There are three main causes of tooth wear:

- **Erosion** The dissolution of teeth by acid, which is mainly present in fruits and drinks. Acids are also present in the stomach, and people who suffer from frequent regurgitation or from the eating disorder bulimia nervosa also show a characteristic pattern of erosion.
- **Attrition** The physical wearing down of teeth by contact with opposing teeth, caused by eating or grinding.
- **Abrasion** The physical wearing down of teeth by other factors, most commonly toothbrushes.

In most cases, at least two or all three factors contribute to worn teeth in any individual. The dentist has to identify and remove the causes.

Harmful agents

The mouth and teeth are at daily risk from a variety of factors, but regular and efficient cleaning can prevent problems. Accurate figures for the incidence of some conditions can be difficult to ascertain, because some people rarely or never see a dentist.

tooth decay

infections

gum disease

age and wear

SUPPORTING STRUCTURE DISORDERS

The "supporting structures" of the teeth are the gingiva (gums) and the bone and periodontal ligaments that hold and support the teeth in the jaws. The bacteria in dental plaque cause inflammation of these tissues, first affecting the gums (gingivitis) before spreading to destroy the supporting bone and ligaments of the periodontium (periodontal disease).

When the inflammation is limited to the gums, the condition is reversible by more effective tooth brushing to remove plaque. The disorder becomes irreversible once the bone has been affected.

Periodontal diseases actually consist of a number of different disorders that tend to be categorized according to how fast they progress. Chronic periodontitis is the most common form of the disease, which advances at different rates in different people but tends to progress slowly, with occasional periods of rapid progression. Chronic periodontitis can be diagnosed as early as 13 or 14 years of age, which means that if left untreated, the disease may lead to tooth loss in middle age.

Not all periodontal diseases progress slowly, however. Aggressive periodontitis

LESS COMMON

ORAL CANCER
There are 30,000 new cases of oral cancer every year in the U.S.; more than 8,000 people will die of it.

is a condition that predominantly affects adolescents and young adults and can lead to tooth loss at a much earlier age. One very aggressive, and fortunately very rare, type of periodontal disease is seen in children and affects the primary teeth, although the permanent teeth may later become involved as well. Some rare syndromes are also linked with aggressive periodontitis in the very young.

ALLERGIC REACTIONS

An allergy to a food, a bite or sting, or a specific medication can lead to a swollen tongue, causing breathing difficulties. Some people are allergic to some of the products used in dentistry, such as dental amalgam, and to materials used in crown and denture manufacture.

DEVELOPMENTAL DISORDERS

Clefts of the lip and palate occur when the lips or the bones of the roof of the mouth fail to fuse properly during development. These clefts may be present either on their own or in combination. Clefts are now managed very successfully by teams of hospital-based specialists.

There is considerable developmental variation in the numbers of teeth. There may be extra (or supplemental) teeth or too few—a condition known as hypodontia.

The position and growth of the jaws can also vary, and this affects the position of the teeth. Malocclusion refers to any degree of irregular contact of the teeth of the upper jaw with the teeth of the lower jaw, including overbites. About 90 percent of schoolchildren have some malocclusion, but only 10 to 15 percent require treatment. Although there are no specific guidelines for deciding how much misalignment is too much, treatment is carried out if it causes problems with the child's bite, speech, or appearance.

TRAUMA

The teeth and the jaws are both at risk from trauma. Teeth can be chipped or literally knocked out of the mouth. Occasionally, a tooth may suffer a fracture of the root, which may cause the tooth to become mobile. The site, extent, and direction of the fracture can only be confirmed by X ray.

Trauma can also lead to a fracture of the jaw, which again depends on the site to which the force is applied. Fractures of the jaws are most commonly sustained during sports, falls, and fights.

When participating in contact sports, protection—including helmets with grills across the mouth and plastic mouth guards—should be worn at all times. In vehicles, seat belts should always be used and crash helmets or cycle helmets should be worn by cyclists and motorcyclists.

INFECTIONS

Although caused primarily by bacteria, dental caries is rarely, if ever, referred to as an infection. Gingivitis and periodontal disease are often known as indigenous infections, because they are caused by a buildup of bacteria that are already present in the mouth. Both periodontal disease and caries can lead to the formation of abscesses, localized infections caused by the buildup of pus. In some cases, local infections can develop and spread, causing osteomyelitis, an infection of the bones of the jaw.

Does periodontal disease increase the risk of developing heart disease?

There is some recent evidence to suggest that people with periodontal disease may be at increased risk of developing heart problems. One explanation for this link might be through bacteria from the mouth being able to get into the bloodstream and cause inflammation in the blood vessels in the heart. Some individuals, however, might be at risk from both heart disease and periodontal disease because of factors that predispose to these diseases: poor diet, smoking, and perhaps stress. Much more research needs to be carried out before any clear causal links between these two very common diseases can be established.

ASK THE EXPERT

The most common viral infection that affects the mouth is the cold sore (herpes labialis). This is caused by the herpes simplex virus and usually occurs during periods of stress or when a person is recovering from illness. Other less-common viral infections that can affect the mouth include shingles (herpes zoster), chicken pox (varicella) and hand, foot, and mouth disease (coxsackie virus). Fungal infections (candidiasis) that occur beneath dentures are also quite common and can be difficult to treat. Candidiasis (oral thrush) often occurs in babies' mouths.

TUMORS

Growths of abnormal cells, or tumors, in the mouth may be benign or malignant. Benign tumors include fibromas, which are small fibrous lumps that may appear on the tongue or gums and lipomas, which contain mainly fat. Adenomas, or glandular tumors, may also occur in the salivary glands. Benign tumors rarely cause adverse symptoms and can be removed surgically, particularly if there is any suspicion that they may be malignant or if they are growing quickly.

Malignant tumors also affect the mouth. The most common type is squamous cell carcinoma, which grows from the surface layers of epithelial cells that line the mouth. Malignant disease can spread to other parts of the body, and early diagnosis and management are essential to maximize the chances of cure.

Who's who—meet the dental experts

Dental care is a team effort. During any one visit to the dentist's office, a patient may be seen by more than one professional. There are also specialists whose expertise may be needed.

DENTIST

Licensure requirements in the United States vary by state. The majority of dentists (dental surgeons) are able to provide a wide range of dental treatment including extractions, fillings, crowns, bridges, dentures, and cleaning. Dentists are also permitted to carry out treatment on patients who are under sedation.

From time to time, a dentist may consider that some of the treatment a patient needs is quite complex and demands additional experience. Under these circumstances, the dentist may refer the patient to a specialist such as an orthodontist or periodontist.

DENTAL HYGIENIST

The dental hygienist undertakes a wide range of duties that complement the work of the dentist to maintain dental health. The hygienist is principally involved with providing dental health education to patients, as well as cleaning the teeth when necessary. They are able to place sealants on the surfaces of the back teeth to help prevent the development of dental caries. Hygienists may take impressions (molds) of the teeth to make plaster models, to replace crowns (caps) that have fallen off, and to place temporary fillings in teeth in which the permanent fillings have been lost.

ORTHODONTIST

Orthontics is a separate dental profession in the United States. An orthodontist specializes in the diagnosis, prevention, and treatment of facial and dental irregularities. This speciality requires training in the design, application, and control of corrective appliances, often braces, to bring teeth, lips, and jaws into alignment. All orthodontists are dentists, but only about 6 percent of dentists are orthodontists.

DENTAL TECHNICIAN

Dental technicians work either in large, commercial laboratories or, very occasionally, in smaller laboratories

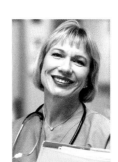

ORAL/MAXILLOFACIAL SURGEON

Oral and maxillofacial surgeons are dentists who have undergone further training to specialize in surgery to the face, mouth, and jaws. They can treat problems that affect the biting function and appearance of the teeth and jaws. Extracting wisdom teeth, straightening misaligned jaws, and offering reconstructive surgery after tumor removal, for example, are all undertaken by an oral or maxillofacial surgeon.

linked to particular dental practices. Their role is to make the crowns, bridges, dentures, and other restorations that the dentist fits in the mouth.

PERIODONTIST

If gum problems are severe, a dentist may refer a patient to a periodontist, who specializes in the diagnosis, prevention, and treatment of periodontal (gum) diseases and in the placement of dental implants. This specialty requires years of training after dental school, as does orthodontics..

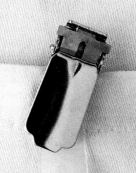

FINDING OUT WHAT IS WRONG

Although a dentist may need X-ray confirmation of suspected problems, most conditions of the mouth and teeth are clearly visible to the naked eye and are easily diagnosed. Routine dental checkups—the mainstay of oral health—are painless and do not take much time.

The dental examination

A routine dental checkup requires an appointment of approximately 15 minutes and will involve a clinical examination. X rays may be taken if required.

A dental examination will follow the same format regardless of whether you are visiting your regular dentist or seeing a dentist for the first time. The dentist will begin by asking you questions about any dental problems or symptoms that you might have before checking on your more general health.

LOOKING OUTSIDE THE MOUTH

When you walk into the dentist's office, the dentist will be looking for any signs that might be relevant to your medical or dental health. For example,
- Do you appear pale and particularly anxious?
- Are you out of breath?
- Do you have any noticeable lumps or swellings on the face or neck?

A more specific extraoral examination can often reveal important information that relates to problems and symptoms that originate inside the mouth. This might involve the dentist palpating
- lumps or swellings;
- lymph glands under the chin and in the neck; or
- jaw joints, ligaments, and muscles that open the mouth.

Cover up
Dentists wear latex gloves—discarded after each patient – to protect both themselves and their patients from blood and saliva-borne pathogens. Increasingly, dentists and their patients are wearing eye protection to guard against harmful airborne particles.

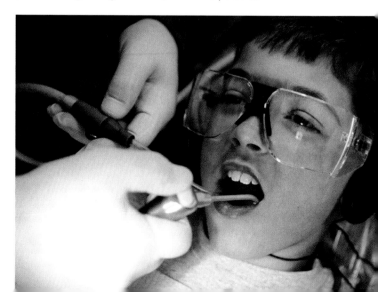

HELP YOUR DENTIST HELP YOU

Describing your general health

When you visit your dentist for a checkup, he or she will already have a record of your general health, but it is necessary to keep these details up to date. The information may be recorded using a questionnaire or by asking you questions directly. Try to think of responses to the following questions and, if you are taking any drugs (for whatever reasons), write them down on paper and hand the list to your dentist when asked.

- *Has your general health changed since your last visit?*

- *Have you had reason to see your doctor or visit a hospital recently and, if so, why?*

- *Are you taking any medicines or using any ointments either given to you by your doctor or bought directly from the pharmacist?*

If you are visiting a dentist for the first time, you will be asked about a number of diseases or conditions that might influence your dental treatment. The dentist may ask the following questions.

- *Do you have high blood pressure or any other heart problems?*

- *Have you ever had rheumatic fever, hepatitis, or jaundice?*

- *Do you have diabetes?*

- *Do you bleed excessively if you cut yourself?*

- *Do you suffer from hay fever or other allergies?*

- *Do you ever have seizures or fainting episodes?*

- *Have you ever had any other viral infection that might still be transmissible?*

LOOKING INSIDE THE MOUTH

Your dentist will examine the soft tissues to check for any change in appearance or signs of disease. The soft tissues cover the floor and roof of the mouth, the lips, the insides of the cheeks, and the gums. The dentist will note whether the soft tissues appear to be dry; this suggests a lack of saliva and possibly poor function of the salivary glands.

The dental chart at your first visit
The dental chart—on paper or computer—is used to record teeth that are affected by dental caries as well as any restorations (fillings, crowns, or bridges) that are present. Each tooth type and surface is labeled to pinpoint specific sites of interest. Any change in the status of the tooth—a new filling or crown, for example—is recorded in the top or lower portions of the chart (not shown).

Charting the teeth

The dentist will complete a dental chart of your teeth every time you have a checkup. Observations will be made, working around the upper and then the lower jaw, and recorded on the chart by the dental assistant. Missing teeth are noted and deleted from the chart; a "missing" tooth that has not yet erupted is denoted U/E (unerupted).
- Occlusal (O) back teeth, or incisal (I) front teeth.
- Lingual (L) lower teeth, or palatal (P) upper teeth.
- Facial (F)—the surface facing toward the lips or cheeks.
- Mesial (M)—the surface orientated toward the midline of the dental arch.
- Distal (D)—the surface orientated away from the midline of the dental arch.
- Buccal (B)—the surface of a posterior tooth that faces toward the cheek.

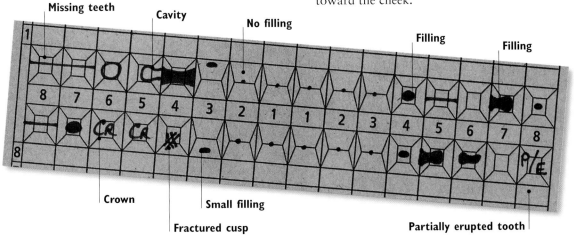

Missing teeth · Cavity · No filling · Filling · Filling

Crown · Small filling · Fractured cusp · Partially erupted tooth

Condition of the gums

The dentist will also check gum (gingival) health, although the status of the bone (periodontium) that supports the teeth can only be assessed using X rays. Simply by looking, the dentist can identify gingivitis, an inflammatory condition leading to swelling of the gums, as well as any areas where the gums appear to be receding from the teeth. When inflammatory disease affects the supporting structures of the teeth, the ligament fibers and bone that hold the teeth in place are resorbed (essentially dissolve away) and a gap opens up between the teeth and the gums. This gap is known as a "pocket," which can be measured in millimeters with an instrument called a periodontal probe and recorded on a pocket chart (sometimes also known as a probing chart).

IMAGING THE TEETH AND THE JAWS

A dentist will usually take an X ray of any tooth or area of the mouth that is causing symptoms to decide the origin and cause of the problem. X rays are also used as part of a routine dental checkup to identify dental caries at sites that may be hard to see and to look for early signs of bone loss around the teeth.

How is it done?

X-ray beams are sent from a radiation source to penetrate structures in the mouth and hit a photographic film that can be placed either inside or outside the mouth.

Most dentists will routinely take four X rays called "bitewings," using small films that are placed inside the mouth. Two films are used for the right side of the jaw and two for the left. These are taken with the patient sitting down.

Some dentists take a panoramic X ray, which uses a much larger film. The patient stands still and the X-ray unit swings around his or her head. The panoramic view provides the dentist with an excellent screening examination of the whole mouth.

What do they show?

Bitewings show radiographic detail of the premolar and molar teeth and enable the dentist to see an image of dental caries and any early loss of bone as a result of periodontal disease. Panoramic films show a much wider view that includes the following:

- All the erupted teeth and the jaws.
- Dental decay, although this may be less obvious than when seen on small films, including bitewings.
- Any teeth that have yet to erupt and their present positions—this is particularly useful in children who may have many teeth that have yet to "come through."
- The position of wisdom teeth that may be unable to erupt because they are growing into the teeth in front (impacted).
- The level of the bone around the teeth in both jaws.
- Any abscesses or cysts associated with the teeth or jaws.

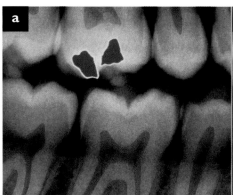 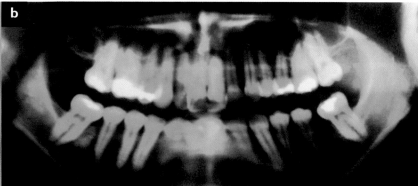

Bitewing and panoramic radiographs

a Bitewing X rays give an early indication of caries forming between the teeth. This X ray also shows two fillings in an upper molar (dark shapes). The pulp of each tooth, which contains blood vessels, is false-colored pink.

Levels of bone between the teeth are clearly picked up on the X ray and can be assessed by the dentist.

b A false-color panoramic X ray shows the teeth and surrounding structures on one film, taken as the

camera swings around from one side of the jaw to the other. Cysts, impacted or unerupted teeth, fractures, and tumors that invade bone will all be visible on this type of X ray; the bright areas in the crowns of the teeth are fillings.

CURRENT TREATMENTS

Dentists have a wide range of treatment options when dealing with teeth and gum problems. More sophisticated approaches to pain relief and anxiety-lowering medications mean that even complicated dental procedures are now carried out safely and with minimal discomfort.

Drugs in dentistry

The range of drugs available to aid dental treatment is more sophisticated than ever before, and many disorders can now be cured with a short course of medication. Other conditions require lifelong treatment with support from a range of specialists.

DENTAL ANESTHESIA

Most dental procedures are carried out under some form of local anesthesia so that any accompanying sensation of pain is eliminated and treatment can be completed in the shortest possible time.

Freezing the gum

Local anesthetics are drugs given by injection to numb the teeth that are undergoing treatment. This is probably the part of dentistry that the majority of people find most uncomfortable, although topical anesthetic creams are available to apply to the site where the injection is to be given. In the upper jaw, the injection is given next to the tooth or teeth receiving treatment so only a small area is anesthetized. In the lower jaw, the injection is given at the back of the mouth to anesthetize the main nerve trunk. This means that all of the teeth,

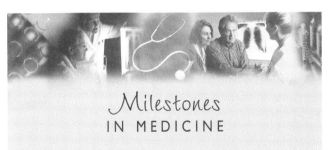

Milestones
IN MEDICINE

Alcohol and opium had been used to combat the pain of surgery, but the first recorded use of anesthesia in dentistry was in Hartford, Connecticut, in 1844. Dentist Horace Wells—under the influence of nitrous oxide ("laughing") gas—had a tooth pulled by a colleague. Two years later, Wells's former partner used ether successfully. Cocaine was also used in the 19th century, until its addictive properties became known. The cocaine substitute Novocain was synthesized in 1905; injections of the drug and its derivatives are still used as local anesthetics for dental procedures.

gums and lower lip on one side of the mouth become numb. The most commonly used local anesthetic drug will work effectively for more than an hour to allow the dentist to complete the treatment.

General anesthetics

General anesthetics achieve complete anesthesia by putting the patient to sleep. They also contain drugs that relax the muscles. For a patient in the hospital, premedication drugs are used to help relieve anxiety, promote amnesia, relax the vocal cords, and reduce the amount of saliva in the mouth. The general anesthetic is then started by injecting the drug into a vein. This acts very quickly, and the anesthesia is then maintained by breathing nitrous oxide gas.

General anesthetics can also be given to outpatients who are allowed to go home the same day after a short period of recovery. These patients are mostly children who require a number of teeth to be extracted and who may be too young to tolerate injections. In these cases, nitrous oxide gas is used as the main drug to achieve anesthesia for the short time needed to extract the teeth. Also, some dentists in the United States specialize in treating patients under general anesthesia in the dentist's own office.

ON THE CUTTING EDGE

Vaccines to protect against dental caries

Because dental caries is such a problem, efforts have been made to develop an anticaries vaccine. Proteins from the surface of the bacterium that causes caries—*Streptococcus mutans*—have been injected into animals and found to elevate the number of protective antibodies produced against caries. Whole bacteria have also been used in human volunteers who swallowed the cells, which then stimulated immune tissue to release antibodies. Another method tested involves using antibodies against the enzyme the bacteria use to make the sticky substance (called glucan) that helps them stick to teeth.

Although work on caries vaccines has been underway for many years, more research is needed before a safe and effective vaccine can be introduced for widespread use in humans.

DENTAL SEDATION

Nitrous oxide can also be used to sedate adult or child patients who are particularly anxious about dental treatment. A sedated patient will be much less anxious about treatment and can still communicate with the dentist throughout. Intravenous sedatives can also be used in adults to great effect. The most common drug in current use is midazolam, which has the benefit of inducing both relaxation and amnesia at the same time.

TREATING TOOTHACHE

Analgesics are used at some time by the majority of the population to relieve the symptoms of pain associated with dental disease, usually toothache. Aspirin and acetaminophen will both help relieve dental pain, although the permanent resolution of symptoms will only be achieved when the cause of the pain has been addressed, so a visit to a dentist is still necessary.

Aspirin has the effect of "thinning the blood" and prolonging the time that a person is likely to bleed after a cut or tooth extraction. It is therefore very important that the dentist is informed if a patient has taken aspirin, even if it is just one or two tablets, in an attempt to relieve pain. If a tooth is extracted, bleeding from the gums may be more prolonged and difficult to stop without the use of stitches.

Acetaminophen, in addition to relieving pain, has the effect of reducing body temperature. It can be given in liquid form to young children who are suffering from teething pain.

INFECTIONS

Antibiotics or antimicrobials are used to treat bacterial infections such as dental abscesses. It is absolutely vital that the dentist be able to treat the cause of the abscess, and this might mean that a tooth requires root canal therapy or extraction.

Some dental infections such as herpes and candidiasis are caused by viruses or fungi, and in these cases, antibiotics will be of very little, if any, use. Antiviral or antifungal drugs might be needed.

It is important to remember that all drugs have side effects as well as beneficial actions, and it is essential that you tell your dentist if you have had any sort of "reaction" to a drug in the past. This will help the dentist choose the most appropriate and safest drug to give you for any specific problem or treatment.

Drilling and filling

Even though there have been considerable improvements in dental health over the last 30 years, restoring teeth that have been affected by tooth decay or extensive wear is still one of the main challenges facing today's dentists.

Fillings may be required for a number of reasons:
- to replace part of a tooth affected by dental caries;
- to replace old fillings that have deteriorated;
- to repair teeth that have been accidentally chipped, cracked or fractured;
- to repair teeth that have worn extensively.

TREATING DECAYED TEETH

The first task is to remove all of the dental caries from the tooth. If caries has redeveloped beneath an old filling, the filling has to be removed first so that the decay can be seen and eliminated. The dentist is aiming to make a cavity that is disease-free and clean and will hold a filling for many years. Traditionally, this has meant cutting away extra tooth tissue that might have been weakened by the removal of the decay and also ensuring that the cavity has undercuts so that the filling will not fall out. Together, the filling and the remains of the tooth must be strong enough to withstand all of the normal forces of biting and eating.

Diamonds are forever
A colored scanning electron micrograph (SEM) of a diamond-tipped dental drill drilling into a tooth. This is carried out to remove decayed or damaged areas of tooth in preparation for a dental filling.

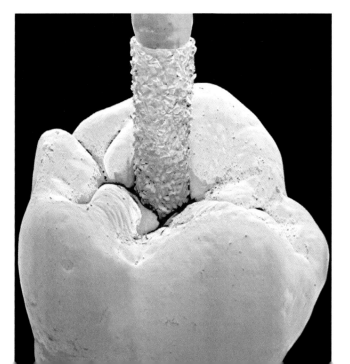

How long should fillings last?

If all the decay is removed from the tooth and the filling is placed with due care and attention, amalgam fillings can last for 20 years or more. One of the problems with any filling is that the edges between the filling and the tooth tend to break down and leave a gap; this is called marginal leakage. The amalgam actually corrodes in the mouth but the products of the corrosion help fill any small gaps that form between the filling and the tooth.

Even crowns don't last forever. All crowns have an edge that meets the tooth, and this is at risk from decay and eventual breakdown. If the dentist keeps this edge above the gum, it will be easier to clean, which may increase the longevity of the restoration.

ASK THE EXPERT

Extra retention

When the amount of tooth that remains is insufficient to hold a filling, it will be necessary to try to get extra retention for the filling. For many years, this has been achieved by drilling small pins into the tooth to act as retaining posts for the filling material. Dental materials, especially those used at the front of the mouth, can also be bonded to the teeth. This requires "treating" the tooth surface first with an acid to etch away part of the highly mineralized surface so that it becomes more irregular and better able to hold a filling. Bonding resins are available to help glue the filling material to the tooth surface, and this technique can be used to build up and restore teeth that have worn down.

New materials, new methods

The development of glues and resins to bond fillings to teeth brought with it a change in the traditional approach of drilling large cavities and removing excessive amounts of healthy tooth substance to retain fillings.

Now, the aim is still to remove all of the tooth tissue damaged by dental caries but no more—as much as possible of the natural tooth is retained. A plastic resin can also be bonded to seal other areas on the tooth that might be at risk from dental caries in the future.

FILLING MATERIALS

The most common filling materials used by dentists are
- Dental amalgam, which is mainly used to fill back teeth.
- Composites, which are tooth-colored resins containing small glass particles—for extra hardness and resistance. They are used only for filling front teeth.
- Glass ionomers, which adhere to the tooth structure and are believed to have an effect in inhibiting dental decay.
- Compomers, which are a mixture of a glass ionomer and an acrylic resin to give extra strength and resistance to wear. The appearance is better than that of glass ionomers.

INLAYS

Inlays are restorations that are made by preparing the cavity in the tooth in much the same way as for a routine filling, but then the dentist takes an impression (mold) of the cavity so that the dental technician has a plaster model that can be used in making the inlay in the laboratory. Traditionally, inlays have been made out of gold mixed with other metals, but they are now available in tooth-colored composite and porcelain. Gold inlays are wear-resistant, strong, and very long-lasting, but their construction is technically demanding and requires a high level of skill from both the dentist and the technician.

Is dental amalgam safe?

TALKING POINT

Dentists have used dental amalgam for more than 100 years. However, some countries have stopped its use because of concerns over its safety. Amalgam contains mercury, and there are worries that this might be released when the amalgam is placed in the mouth and when old amalgam fillings are removed. There is no firm evidence linking the use of amalgam to general medical problems, except in the case of allergy, and the FDA supports its use, citing extensive studies and recommendation by the World Health Organization. Amalgam remains an excellent filling material that resists wear and is cheap and easy to use.

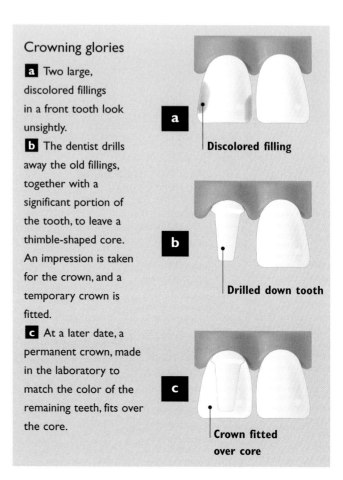

Crowning glories
a Two large, discolored fillings in a front tooth look unsightly.
b The dentist drills away the old fillings, together with a significant portion of the tooth, to leave a thimble-shaped core. An impression is taken for the crown, and a temporary crown is fitted.
c At a later date, a permanent crown, made in the laboratory to match the color of the remaining teeth, fits over the core.

a | Discolored filling

b | Drilled down tooth

c | Crown fitted over core

CROWNS

Crowns, or caps, are restorations that are usually made to fit over a tooth that has been cut, trimmed, or filed down by the dentist. Crowns are needed if dental caries has been extensive and the resulting filling is so large that the remaining tooth is weak and likely to fracture. The crown holds or splints the filling and remaining tooth together. Crowns on back teeth are made of gold and other metals. Crowns at the front of the mouth always have a porcelain face but may have a metal core for added strength.

VENEERS

Veneers are used for discolored front teeth: The tooth may have died and had the nerve removed or a long-term stain cannot be removed by polishing the tooth surface.

A small layer of the outer-facing enamel surface of the tooth is filed away and a mold is taken. A very thin shell of porcelain is made to cover the filed surface and bonded onto the remaining enamel of the tooth surface. The thin shell of porcelain is delicate to work with but gains strength once it has been bonded to the tooth.

Orthodontic treatment

Orthodontics is the branch of dentistry concerned with correcting irregularities in the position of the teeth. For increasing numbers of children, orthodontics may be the first real experience with prolonged dental treatment.

Orthodontics is concerned with the growth of the face and jaws, the development of the teeth, and the correction of positional problems with the teeth as they arise. This may involve just one or two teeth or it may extend to the majority of teeth in both jaws. Possible problems include

- too few teeth being present;
- too many teeth being present;
- teeth that develop in the wrong position;
- too much space between teeth;
- teeth that don't meet properly when bitten together;
- upper front teeth that protrude in front of the lower teeth; and
- lower front teeth that bite in front of the upper teeth.

THE ROLE OF THE DENTIST

All dentists play a role in the diagnosis of problems associated with the development and growth of the jaws and teeth. The first signs of problems can be seen as early as 7 or 8 years of age, which is a good reason for ensuring that children visit the dentist regularly. The dentist can check the order in which the primary teeth are lost and permanent teeth erupt, how the jaws grow in relation to each other, and the form and position of

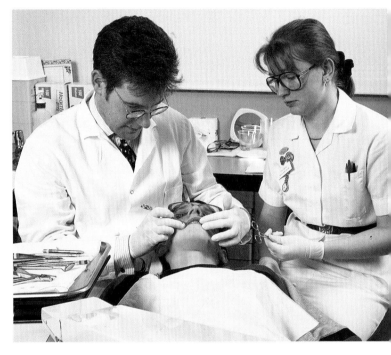

Checking progress
A boy's fixed braces are checked by an orthodontist and assistant to monitor the progress of the treatment and the condition of the adjustable wire and to check for any rubbing in the mouth.

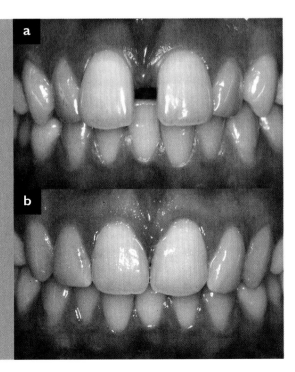

Closing the gap

a A young patient is brought in for orthodontic treatment to close the gap between the two front teeth—both for cosmetic purposes and to improve the biting functions of the front teeth.

b After braces have been worn for 18 months, the gap between the two front teeth has closed and the other teeth are more regularly aligned.

the permanent teeth. The dentist will also recognize when referral to an orthodontic specialist is required.

The specialist

An orthodontist will undertake a more detailed examination using X rays, photographs, and models of the teeth and jaws and will also look at the position of the teeth in relation to the skull bones. Once any problems have been identified, a plan of action can be developed. In some cases, the specialist will carry out the treatment; in others, detailed treatment instructions will be passed to the dentist.

TREATMENT DECISIONS

The decision on whether treatment should go ahead is a matter for discussion among the child, parents, and the specialist or dentist. The discussion should focus on the potential risks, as well as the benefits. There are two main reasons for carrying out orthodontic treatment:

• To improve appearance.
• To improve dental health, enabling the patient to function better when biting and eating.

Treatment should be contemplated only when it is going to benefit one, or perhaps both, of these features. Indeed, a patient may think that the time and effort required for orthodontic treatment may not justify the perceived benefit. If, after discussion of all the issues, some doubts remain, it is probably wise not to continue.

Most orthodontic treatment is undertaken in children at the time when the last primary teeth are being lost and the permanent teeth have erupted, usually around 12 to 14 years of age. In younger children, recommended treatment may have to be deferred until more teeth erupt. Occasionally, carefully planned extractions of one or more primary teeth might prevent a problem from developing in the first place. Conversely, some problems may become more difficult to manage successfully if left for too long.

BRACED FOR BRACES

The primary orthodontic tool used to adjust tooth position is the orthodontic appliance, or brace. Because successful tooth movement can be achieved only gradually, these are often worn for 2 to 3 years. There are three main types of dental brace:

• **Fixed appliances** These are made up of several small brackets or bands, which are bonded (glued) to the teeth and then joined together using a combination of wires and very small elastic bands that apply the force for moving teeth. The fixed appliance cannot be removed from the mouth by the patient.

IT'S NOT TRUE!

"Orthodontic treatment can only be carried out in children"

Many orthodontic problems can be corrected in adults, who often make well-motivated and compliant patients. Potential problems caused by crowded teeth can be avoided by timely treatment, using tooth removal or braces. By adulthood, however, the growth of the jaws is virtually complete. This means that irregular tooth positions resulting from a significant discrepancy in the size of the jaw can only be corrected by surgically altering the relationship between the jaws.

• **Removable appliances** These can be removed from the mouth for cleaning. They have a plastic base covering the roof of the mouth, metal clasps that hold the brace in the mouth, and springs that apply the force required to move the teeth in the desired direction.
• **Functional appliances** These devices are bulky and may have a headgear component outside the mouth. They apply, modify, or eliminate the forces generated by the muscles and jaws during growth. They can only be used for growing children.

The surgical approach

Occasionally, surgical correction to the jaw is undertaken in young adults when jaw development is complete. This involves a team of specialists.

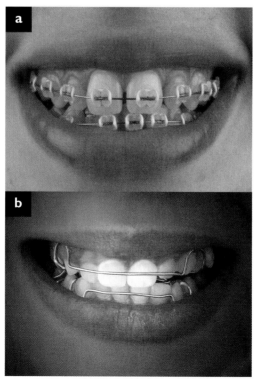

Fixed and removable braces
a *Fixed braces are worn to correct poor alignment between upper and lower jaws or overcrowding of teeth.*
b *Removable braces (retainers) are worn when teeth misalignment is minor or after the removal of fixed braces used to correct a major misalignment.*

Root canal therapy

When pulp death occurs, either through extensive decay or trauma or rarely through irritation from dental filling materials, the dentist's options are extraction or root canal therapy. This involves replacing the pulp of the tooth with a gutta percha—a resinous gum—filling.

When dental caries becomes extensive, bacteria can migrate through the remaining dentin to cause inflammation of the pulp, the central tissue of the tooth containing the blood and nerve supply. This is likely to cause severe toothache, which if untreated can last for a considerable time. Eventually, the inflammation becomes irreversible, the pulp tissue dies, and the infection may spread to form an abscess at the end of the root.

At this stage, removal of the decay and placement of a filling will not solve the problem.

The dentist might use a hot or very cold stimulus to see whether there is any feeling left in the tooth. Alternatively, an electric instrument can be used to determine whether there is any living tissue left. A gentle tap to the tooth will check for tenderness—a possible sign of an abscess, although an X ray will be required to confirm this.

THE RUBBER TENT

Before starting root canal treatment, the dentist will place a sheet of rubber over the tooth and then stretch it out so that the tooth becomes isolated in the mouth. This is done for two main reasons:

• To try to make sure that saliva doesn't get into the tooth and contaminate the root canal.
• To prevent any small instruments or materials from being swallowed or damaging the gums around the tooth being worked on.

TREATING THE ROOT CANAL

The first step in treatment is to remove any decay and to drill through the remaining part of the tooth into the top of the central chamber of the pulp. The inflamed or dead pulp tissue can then be removed, and saline is used to flush out any debris that remains. Small files are used to clean the walls of the "canals" in the roots of the teeth. The dentist has to be certain that all the debris and any signs of infection have been removed before placing any filling in the root canal.

The clean canal is filled, usually with long fine cones of gutta percha, which is introduced into the canals using fine, thin instruments. The gutta percha is sealed in place using a paste (sealant) that fills the tiny space between the gutta percha and the side of the canal walls. The aim is to fill and seal the entire length of the root canal.

WHAT HAPPENS NEXT?

The next step depends on the amount of tooth left behind. If most of the tooth is still intact, the dentist can insert a conventional filling to fill the cavity; the tooth is then likely to last for many years. If there is little natural tooth left, it might be necessary to remove some of the root filling and make a mold of the space created in the root canal. Using a plaster model of the tooth created from the mold, the dental technician can make a metal post and core. The post is glued into the canal with the metal core protruding beyond the root. The technician can then make a crown to fit over the core to restore the tooth.

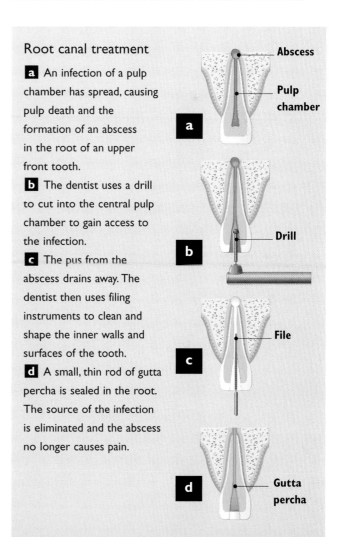

Root canal treatment

a An infection of a pulp chamber has spread, causing pulp death and the formation of an abscess in the root of an upper front tooth.

b The dentist uses a drill to cut into the central pulp chamber to gain access to the infection.

c The pus from the abscess drains away. The dentist then uses filing instruments to clean and shape the inner walls and surfaces of the tooth.

d A small, thin rod of gutta percha is sealed in the root. The source of the infection is eliminated and the abscess no longer causes pain.

Abscess
Pulp chamber
a
Drill
b
File
c
Gutta percha
d

Replacing missing teeth

Teeth may be lost through trauma, but more often they are lost to decay. There are several ways in which dentists can replace missing teeth after tooth extraction: by creating a bridge, by implanting one or more false teeth, or by using dentures.

Not all teeth need to be replaced after extraction. Research has shown that nobody needs all 32 teeth to eat properly. Indeed, it is possible to function perfectly well with just 21 teeth at the front of the mouth: 10 upper and 10 lower. When a tooth is extracted from the front of the mouth, however, most people are understandably anxious to have the gap filled as quickly as possible.

IMMEDIATE REPLACEMENT OF TEETH

When the loss of a front tooth is planned in advance, the dentist will ensure that the space is filled immediately after the extraction. The easiest way to do this is by using a small denture or, if a denture is already present, by adding an extra false tooth to the existing denture. This method will necessitate a visit to the dentist before the tooth is extracted so that molds of the teeth can be taken to make the denture. Of course, if the tooth is being extracted because of an emergency, this preliminary visit may not be possible and the patient may have to accept a gap in the teeth for a short period of time.

The so-called "immediate denture" is often neither the best nor a long-term replacement, particularly for a single tooth, but its use does allow the dentist and the patient to discuss treatment options that may be used in due course: a bridge, implant, or permanent palate.

DENTAL IMPLANTS

Dental implants have been around for many years, but only relatively recently have techniques and materials been perfected to the extent that the use of dental implants has become more common. Implants are sometimes referred to as "screw-in" teeth.

Things to know about dental implants

- An implant is essentially a rod of titanium that is screwed into the jaw. This is then covered with a crown or used as part of the support for a bridge or palate.
- The surface of the implant bonds to or integrates with the bone of the jaw—this is known as osseointegration.
- One implant can be used to support a single crown, whereas multiple implants are needed to support bridges or dentures.
- The process of inserting implants is undertaken in two stages: first, a surgical treatment to screw in the implant(s), and second, a dental treatment to make the final restoration that fits over the implant.
- Implants must be looked after very carefully by maintaining good oral hygiene. It is not always easy to remove an implant if the need arises.
- Implants can be done under a local anesthetic; there may be discomfort or pain once this wears off.
- The provision of implants is a specialty service and is therefore expensive.

Bridges

A bridge spans a gap of one—or two—missing teeth. In bridgework, a false tooth is attached to the surrounding teeth, which must be in good condition. In preparation, these are reduced in size to accommodate a crown; these act as anchors for the false tooth. While the porcelain bridge is being made, a temporary plastic bridge will be in place. It will have a pontic (false tooth) to replace the missing tooth. The final porcelain bridge will only be fixed in place once it has been fitted and the color, shape, and size are correct.

In recent years, significant advances have been made in the development of "gluelike" resins and the techniques by which metals can be stuck onto tooth surfaces with minimal, if any, cutting of the tooth surface. This means that dental technicians can now make "stick-on bridges," which the dentist simply sticks onto the teeth. These resin-bonded bridges are very useful for gaps at the front of the mouth.

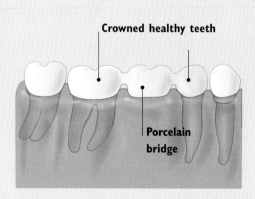

Crowned healthy teeth

Porcelain bridge

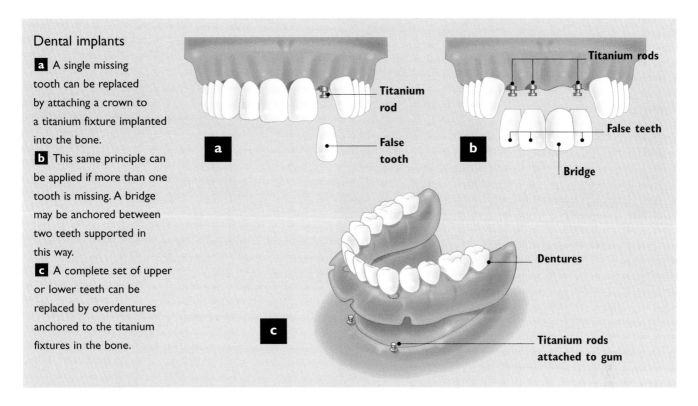

Dental implants

a A single missing tooth can be replaced by attaching a crown to a titanium fixture implanted into the bone.

b This same principle can be applied if more than one tooth is missing. A bridge may be anchored between two teeth supported in this way.

c A complete set of upper or lower teeth can be replaced by overdentures anchored to the titanium fixtures in the bone.

a — Titanium rod — False tooth

b — Titanium rods — False teeth — Bridge

c — Dentures — Titanium rods attached to gum

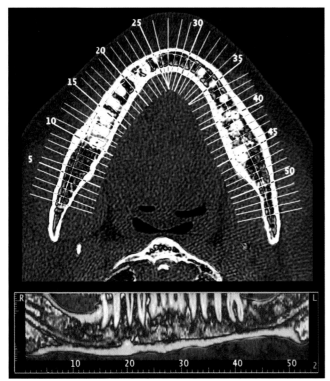

Planning implant surgery
The bone has to be strong enough to maintain dental implants, so CT scans are taken prior to surgery. The top scan shows the jaw and teeth (white). In the lower scan, the teeth appear blue and the bone orange. In this case, the bone was deemed too fragile for implants.

FITTING A DENTURE

When some natural teeth remain and a denture is used to fill the gaps, it is often referred to as a "palate" or "plate." These partial dentures can be made to replace any number of teeth in the jaw. They are made of acrylic resin or a combination of acrylic resin on a metal base (which is a mixture of chrome and cobalt). When the remaining natural teeth are in good condition, they can be used to provide support for the partial denture. Clasps are used to clip around the teeth, although if these are used on natural teeth at the front of the mouth, they may appear unsightly. A compromise then has to be made between appearance and how secure the palate is in the mouth.

Partial denture
Partial dentures can be fixed or removable and support one or more missing teeth in a jaw. They are retained in the mouth either by the underlying tissues or by wires attached to the remaining teeth. The denture here holds two false teeth (2nd and 3rd from right).

Wire attached to healthy teeth

False teeth

IT'S NOT TRUE!

"Dentures will be the end of all my problems"

If teeth have been causing a lot of problems and pain, it is natural to want to have them taken out and replaced by dentures. It is wrong, however, to think that all the problems will be solved when the natural teeth have been replaced. The majority of people who have dentures find them difficult to get used to, and when the natural teeth have been extracted, some of the bone of the jaws "dissolves away," so, with time, the dentures become progressively loose. Dentures, like teeth, need to be maintained in good condition, and regular visits to the dentist are still recommended so that any potential gum problems can be identified and managed before symptoms develop.

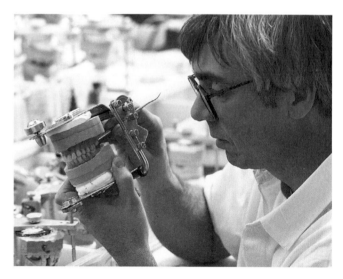

Technical support
Full dentures consist of a plastic base to which ceramic or acrylic teeth are attached. A dental technician makes dentures to fit a molded model of the patient's mouth. A combination of suction and the supporting gums holds the dentures in place.

FALSE TEETH

"False teeth" is the colloquial term for dentures, most often used when all of the natural teeth have been lost and replaced by upper and lower dentures—complete dentures. The transition from natural teeth to dentures is never easy. It is made a little easier, however, when a patient has been losing teeth over a number of years and these teeth have been added to a smaller, partial denture as they are extracted. As this partial denture gets progressively bigger, the adaptation to complete dentures when the last natural teeth are removed is less challenging for the patient. The artificial teeth that are added to the denture are based on earlier molds of the patient's teeth.

It is not always possible to plan such a transition. Some patients may need to have all of the remaining natural teeth extracted during just one or two appointments. In such cases, an immediate denture is used to replace the teeth when they are extracted, although the dentist and the dental technician have to use some "guesswork" because they have not been able to take a mold of the gums without the teeth to make an accurately fitting denture. The immediate denture will need to be replaced in due course, usually in 6 to 12 months at the most.

Smiling with confidence
Dentures can make an enormous difference to a patient's self-esteem, especially if an individual has been in pain from decaying teeth. They are not an instant solution, however, and can take time to feel "natural."

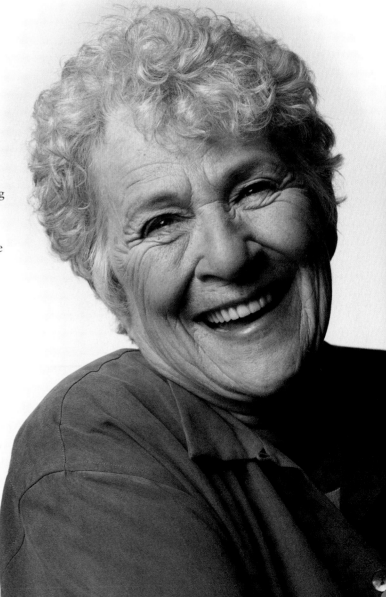

Treating gum diseases

Gingivitis and periodontal disease develop because of inadequate personal oral hygiene and a buildup of dental plaque. Avoiding plaque buildup and promptly removing any that does occur are the cornerstones of treatment.

VISITING THE DENTIST

The dentist or hygienist aims to reduce an individual's risk of gum disease through effective education and through removing any buildup of plaque and calculus.

Improving personal oral hygiene

The first line of treatment is for the hygienist or dentist to spend time trying to find out which teeth, or surfaces of the teeth, are not being brushed effectively. The emphasis, however, is on the patient to improve tooth cleaning in the long term, which often necessitates a significant behavioral change toward improving oral hygiene. The dentist or hygienist has the options of introducing

- a new design of manual toothbrush or perhaps an electric toothbrush;
- a systematic tooth-brushing technique for more thorough cleaning; and
- methods for cleaning between the teeth above and below the gum line such as wood sticks or dental floss.

At successive visits, the dentist or hygienist might measure the amount of plaque on the teeth to ensure that the standard of personal oral hygiene is improving. Areas of plaque buildup may be recorded on a chart for the patient to use as a guide when tooth cleaning.

Scaling and polishing

If there are deposits of calculus on the teeth, they will be removed by the dentist or hygienist because they cannot be removed by tooth brushing alone. When the calculus is above or just below the gum line, it can be seen and removed quite easily by scaling the tooth surfaces. The surfaces are then polished to remove all the deposits of plaque. Cleaning might be carried out using an ultrasonic scaler, which has a metal tip that vibrates at a very high frequency. The scaler has a water spray to cool the tip and impart energy from the fine spray of water bubbles to further enhance tooth cleaning, a process known as ultrasonic cleaning.

With more advanced periodontal disease, the plaque and calculus form on the root surfaces in "pockets" below the gum line. These areas are difficult to clean, because the dentist or hygienist is unable to see the root surface directly

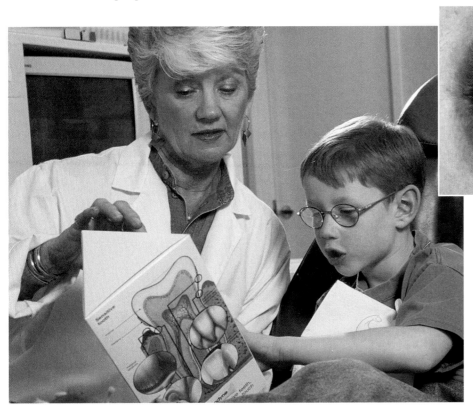

Understanding the basics
As well as removing plaque and calculus, a hygienist also helps patients understand where plaque is likely to build up, perhaps by supplying a chart showing typical buildup patterns to use while brushing, or advising patients to use disclosing tablets, which stain plaque red or blue (above).

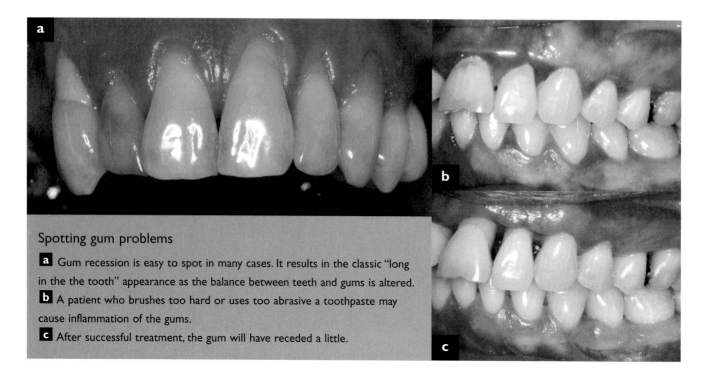

Spotting gum problems

a Gum recession is easy to spot in many cases. It results in the classic "long in the the tooth" appearance as the balance between teeth and gums is altered.
b A patient who brushes too hard or uses too abrasive a toothpaste may cause inflammation of the gums.
c After successful treatment, the gum will have receded a little.

and has to rely on the sense of touch to ensure there are no rough areas of calculus left behind. This procedure is called root planing and is usually carried out under local anesthetic.

THE AIMS OF TREATMENT

An improved standard of oral hygiene and removal of calculus should end inflammation and the gum will shrink and perhaps become reattached to the roots of the teeth. The exposed roots may be sensitive to hot and cold and may also be at risk from dental decay over the long term.

WHEN SURGERY IS NECESSARY

In some cases, the results of scaling and root planing are not as great as hoped. This is often because of a continued failure to improve the standard of oral hygiene. Scaling below the gum line may be impeded by difficult access. The alternative is a surgical procedure, under local anesthetic, that involves making an incision along the gum line and lifting the gum away from the teeth. This allows the dentist to see the calculus deposits directly and considerably improves the access for scaling.

GUM RECESSION

Gum recession can be an alarming development, particularly when it occurs at the front of the mouth, where it can be unattractive. It is essential that the root surface, which is exposed as a result of the gum recession, is kept meticulously clean by effective tooth brushing.

A root exposed through aggressive tooth brushing may become sensitive, decayed, or both. There are special varnishes (with a high fluoride content) and plastic resins that the dentist can apply to harden and desensitize the root surface. This treatment will need to be repeated at regular intervals to be effective.

The appearance of gum recession, even at the front of the mouth, is usually not too obvious, because the lips cover the defect at most times. In more severe cases, however, a specialist might be able to perform a surgical graft to help cover the root by taking a piece of gum from an adjacent tooth or from the roof of the mouth.

OVERGROWTH OF THE GUMS

Some drugs can cause the gums to grow considerably, sometimes so much that the teeth are virtually covered. Such drugs, which are now in common use, include
• **Phenytoin**, which is taken by epileptic patients.
• **Nifedipine**, which is taken to control blood pressure.
• **Cyclosporine**, which is taken to suppress the immune system in patients who have had an organ transplant.
Overgrowth of the gums can be unsightly but can also be surgically corrected under local anesthetic. Unfortunately, there is a high chance of recurrence while the drug is still being taken, although an improvement in personal oral hygiene will lessen this chance. The dentist might consider writing to a patient's doctor or physician to ask whether an alternative drug might be prescribed.

Cancer treatments

Oral cancer has a poor prognosis, often because it is found late. With early diagnosis and treatment, however, its cure rate is more than 90 percent. Its treatment presents a challenge for both the patient and for the multidisciplinary team of experts involved.

Cancer of the mouth (oral cancer) is a rare condition in the U.S. It accounts for about 3% of cancers in men and 2% of cancers in women. It is almost twice as common in men than women, and mostly occurs in people over 45.

Oral cancer, or squamous cell carcinoma, starts in the cells that form the lining of the mouth, on the lips, or on the surface layer covering the tongue. Other cancers that can develop in the mouth area include salivary gland cancer and primary bone cancer, which can develop in the jawbone.

CAUSES AND RISK FACTORS

Those most at risk of developing oral squamous cell carcinomas are smokers and people who drink heavily—and particularly those who do both. Other risk factors include
- pipe smoking and people holding cigarettes between the lips for long periods,
- chewing tobacco or paan,
- "nervous" lip-biting or chewing the inside of the cheek,
- exposure to the sun without adequate SPF protection, causing cancer of the lip.

Most oral cancers are caused by lifestyle rather than any genetically inherited risk of cancer. It is not known what causes salivary gland or primary bone cancer in the jaw.

SYMPTOMS

Early diagnosis is absolutely crucial to the outcome. It is always sensible to have any of the following lesions looked at by a dentist even though, in the majority of cases, they will be harmless:
- A painless ulcer that has been present for more than 2 to 3 weeks and shows no signs of healing.
- Any white patch in the mouth, particularly under the tongue or in the floor of the mouth.
- Any red, inflamed, or swollen areas, especially under the tongue or in the floor of the mouth.

Smoking cigarettes, cigars, or pipes or chewing tobacco is the direct cause of up to 90 percent of oral cancer cases.

A dentist will arrange for such lesions to be seen by a specialist, usually an oral surgeon, who will surgically remove (biopsy) a small part of the affected area, or if it is relatively small, the entire lesion. It will then be examined under a microscope to check for any malignant changes in the cells and tissues.

If the biopsy results indicate cancer, additional tests will be carried out to find out more about the extent (stage) of the cancer. These results will help determine the most appropriate form of treatment.

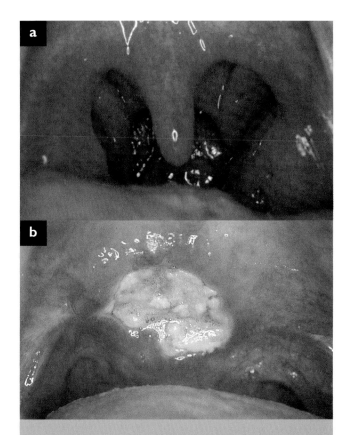

Telltale signs

a In a healthy mouth, tissues are pink and moist. The tonsils on either side of the mouth contain white blood cells to help fight infection.

b Cancerous tissue may show up as white lesions, and for this reason any persistent sores or ulcers should be examined promptly by a doctor or dentist. Treatment is to remove the lesions and is often followed by radiation.

APPROACHES TO TREATMENT

The main types of treatment for cancers of the mouth are surgery and radiation. A team of specialists will decide which form of treatment is best, taking into account factors including age, general health, tumor type, and stage. The team will include these doctors:

- **Oncologist** A specialist in managing cancers, who helps decide on the most appropriate form of treatment.
- **Surgical oncologist (a maxillofacial, plastic, or ENT surgeon)** A surgeon who specializes in mouth and jaw surgery.
- **Radiologist** A doctor who specializes in treating cancers with radiation.
- **Dentist or oral hygienist** Carries out regular checkups and any routine but essential dental care during treatment.
- **Restorative specialist** Provides dentures or implants to replace any teeth or part of the jaw removed during surgery.

- **Dietician** Gives advice regarding dietary issues and any problems with eating.
- **Speech therapist** Helps with speech training after surgical removal of the tumor.

Surgery

Surgical excision of the tumor is almost always necessary. Very small cancers can often be treated with a simple surgical operation under local or general anesthetic, with no need to stay in the hospital overnight. For other cancers, the surgery may need to be more extensive.

In some cases, laser surgery may be used to treat tumors in the mouth. This may be combined with a light-sensitive drug treatment known as photodynamic therapy. Another type of specialty surgery called micrographic surgery is undergoing trials for cancers of the lips and oral cavity. In micrographic surgery, the surgeon not only removes the cancer but also examines the tissue that has been removed under a microscope to check that no cancer cells remain.

Radiation

Radiation may be used alone or after surgery to destroy small areas of cancer that could not be removed.

When radiation therapy is undertaken on the head and neck area, the main salivary glands will almost certainly be affected and the flow of saliva into the mouth reduced considerably. When the mouth dries up—xerostomia (see page 155)—the risk of dental caries increases significantly because of the lack of protective saliva. Synthetic substitutes for natural saliva are available, and these may be applied at regular intervals to help moisten the mouth.

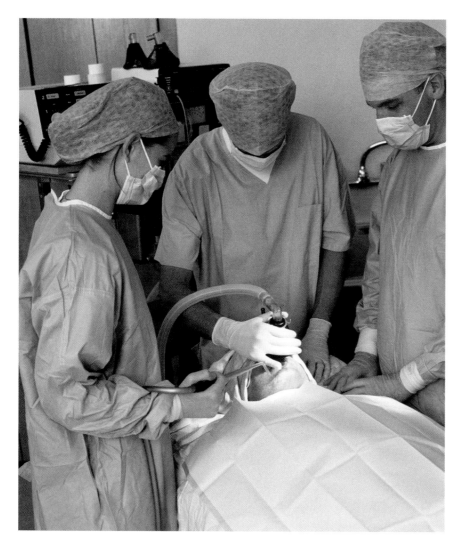

Multidisciplinary team
Surgery for oral cancer involves specialists from many disciplines, with extensive surgery often merely the starting point of treatment. Dental reconstructive work may be necessary once the cancer has been eradicated.

A TO Z
OF DISEASES AND DISORDERS

This section gives information on the main illnesses and medical conditions that affect the eyes and the mouth.

This index is arranged in two alphabetical sections, one for conditions affecting the eyes and one for conditions affecting the mouth. Most entries are structured in a similar way:

What are the causes?

What are the symptoms?

How is it diagnosed?

What are the treatment options?

What is the outlook?

THE EYES

AGE-RELATED MACULAR DEGENERATION (AMD)

The leading cause of irreversible sight loss in Europe and the U.S., this is a progressive wasting of the central part of the retina. There are two types, wet and dry.

What are the causes?

The causes of AMD are not well understood, but advancing age and smoking increase the risk. In dry AMD, changes in the retina take place over a period of years, and a deficiency of antioxidants in one layer of cells in the retina may be a part of the disease process. Thus, a diet rich in antioxidants may have a role in reducing the risk of the disease, although research to support this is still in its early stages. In wet AMD, leaking vessels in the retina cause rapid visual loss.

What are the symptoms?

AMD produces distortion and eventually a loss of the central area of vision. This causes great difficulty in tasks such as reading, recognizing faces, and watching television.

How is it diagnosed?

The doctor makes a diagnosis by looking at the retina and using fluorescein angiography (p. 99). Later in the disease, changes in vision can be picked up by a test in which the patient looks at an Amsler chart, which has grid lines printed on it. A patient with AMD will see distortions of the lines in the center of the chart.

What are the treatment options?

Little can be done to improve the vision of dry AMD sufferers. Wet AMD can sometimes be helped by laser therapy or with an injection of dye in conjunction with laser treatment (this is known as photodynamic therapy, PDT). A low-vision assessment can help the patient make the most of his or her remaining vision.

AMBLYOPIA

Sometimes called a "lazy" eye, amblyopia is poor vision in one eye that is not caused by a defect in the visual pathway and cannot be corrected by lenses.

What are the causes?

Amblyopia can arise in several ways. For example, it may be the result of a big difference in the focusing ability of the two eyes or it can be caused by a squint. In those with amblyopia, the brain gradually learns to ignore the image received from one of the eyes.

What are the symptoms?

The underlying problems that may lead to amblyopia have different signs and symptoms. Failure to treat the underlying problem can result in poor "stereo" vision and depth perception. Often there are no symptoms, which is why testing children's vision before school age is important.

How is it diagnosed?

The conditions that can lead to amblyopia—for example, squints or poor vision in one eye—as well as amblyopia itself are picked up by a routine eye examination. When each eye is tested separately, there will be a substantial difference in the patient's ability to read the standard letter chart. Specific tests for "stereo" vision—the ability to see a three-dimensional image—are used to confirm the diagnosis. Many of these tests are suitable for children. For example, the patient looks at a card or plate, sometimes through special goggles, which shows images that can be seen only by people with good stereoscopic vision.

What are the treatment options?

Exercises that train eye coordination are often combined with lengthy periods of covering the stronger eye with a patch. The earlier the diagnosis, the greater the chance of successful treatment.

ASTIGMATISM

In this condition, which is often inherited, blurred vision is caused by an irregular cornea.

What are the symptoms?

Objects look blurred and distorted because light entering the eye through different parts of the cornea is brought to a focus at different points.

How is it diagnosed?

The optician uses several tests to measure the degree of astigmatism. An instrument called an autorefractor may be used to gain an initial estimate of the patient's condition. As patients look into the autorefractor, they are asked to keep their eyes fixed on a target, such as a balloon, while an estimate of their prescription is made. These initial measurements are refined using a cross-cylinder, which holds two lenses. The patient is asked to compare vision using the two lenses. After checking the patient's response to different lens combinations, the optician will have an accurate picture of the degree of astigmatism in each eye.

What are the treatment options?
Corrective lenses with a cylindrical shape positioned at a certain angle are available in glasses and contact lenses. Refractive surgery is a new alternative.

BASAL CELL CARCINOMA (BCC)
The most common form of cancer, BCC involves the eyelid in about 9 percent of cases.

There are 1 million new cases of basal and squanous cell carcinoma diagnosed every year in the U.S. Basal cell carcinoma is the most common form of skin cancer, accounting for 75 to 90 percent of cases.

There are many complex and potential contributing factors, although the major factor is sun exposure. A lump that grows relatively slowly appears on the surface of the eyelid—usually the lower lid. The diagnosis is confirmed by a biopsy. Small, superficial tumors can be removed by freezing them, but surgery and radiation may be required for larger tumors. If caught early, this cancer has an excellent cure rate.

BLEPHARITIS
Inflammation of the eyelids resulting from an infection, an allergy, or too much glandular secretion.

The edges of the lids become swollen, with crusty deposits around the lashes. An affected eye may be sore, especially in the morning, and red. Treatment will depend on the cause and the severity of the problem. A cleansing solution applied with a cotton swab helps keep the lid clean. Warm compresses of previously boiled water may be soothing and antiallergy drugs or antibiotics may be prescribed.

CATARACT
Misty or blurred vision as a result of loss of transparency in the lens.

What are the causes?
There are various causes of cataracts, most commonly aging, but also injury, diseases such as diabetes, certain drugs, and radiation, such as ultraviolet radiation from the sun. A rare, inherited form can affect newborns; some children develop cataracts as a result of trauma or drugs or with other eye problems such as retinal disease.

What are the symptoms?
Cataracts start small and may not interfere with vision until they are quite large, but even a small cataract can affect daily life if it obscures the central part of the retina. The patient may notice blurred distance and near vision, poor vision at night, and glare from bright lights and reflections. Sometimes they may notice double vision.

How is it diagnosed?
An optician can see a cataract during a routine eye examination. Drops to dilate the pupil to view the cataract clearly may be given on examination.

What are the treatment options?
Cataract is among the most common and treatable eye problems, although treatment is not always necessary and depends on how much the cataract interferes with vision and everyday life. If required, cataract surgery is generally safe and quick (p. 108).

CHALAZION
Chronic inflammation of the gland in the eyelid that produces the oily surface layer of the tear film.

A blockage of the gland causes a gradual swelling on the edge of the eyelid. There may be no symptoms other than the appearance of a lump, but the area may be tender. The appearance of the lump and the surrounding area, as well as the speed of growth and any history, help the correct diagnosis to be made. Some chalazia may disappear spontaneously. Others will gradually disappear with the use of ointment or warm compresses. It may be necessary to cut out the chalazion (see also Hordeolum, p. 140).

COLOR BLINDNESS
An inability to distinguish certain colors; it is extremely rare for a person to have no color vision at all.

What are the causes?
It is estimated that 8 percent of males and 0.5 percent of females are born color-blind. The two most common

forms—protanomaly (weak red vision) and deuteranomaly (weak green vision)—make up 99 percent of all cases.

Most color blindness is genetic, but there are a few types that may develop as a result of damage to the retina or optic nerve. In such cases, the patient may have a different type of color problem in each eye. Inherited color blindness is more common in boys than in girls because the relevant genes occur on the chromosomes that determine gender. Females have two X chromosomes, each carrying the same genes. If there is a defect in a color vision gene on one chromosome, the other can mask its effect. It is only if both copies of the gene carry the defect that a problem becomes apparent. Boys have only one X chromosome, so there is no second copy of the gene to mask a defect.

What are the symptoms?
People with protanomaly see red, orange, yellow, yellow-green, and green all as similar in hue and paler than normal. Those with deuteranomaly find different hues in the green part of the spectrum difficult to distinguish. In some cases, people may be unaware that they have a problem.

How is it diagnosed?
Color blindness can cause learning problems if it is not detected, so early testing is advised. There are specific color tests that involve looking at pictures or plates. The Ishihara test, for example, has colored numbers or patterns set against a different colored background. People with specific color vision defects will see a different number—or no number at all—than those with no defect.

What are the treatment options?
Because color blindness is usually genetic, there is no cure and color cannot be restored. Specially tinted glasses may help some sufferers distinguish colors they find confusing.

COMPUTER-RELATED EYE PROBLEMS
People who use a computer for long periods may experience eye problems such as dryness and headaches.

When people look at a computer screen for a long time, the frequency of blinking slows to just over one third of normal rate, and this can cause the front of the eye to become drier than normal. The problem is compounded when the working area is air-conditioned. People may also experience headaches as a result of focusing at one distance for a long period, from poor lighting or glare from a window nearby, a screen set at the wrong brightness, or from wearing incorrect glasses for the distance to the screen.

Dry eyes can result in itchiness or a gritty sensation in the eye, and symptoms of eye strain may include headaches, sensitivity to light, and red or watery eyes. The eyes may feel "tired" at the end of the day.

An optician can test for visual performance at screen distance and advise on avoiding eye strain or whether a person may need glasses or a different prescription for computer work.

CONJUNCTIVITIS
Inflammation of the outer layer of cells covering the eye.

Conjunctivitis can arise from infection by bacteria or a virus or can be caused by allergy or a toxic reaction. It causes redness of the inner lids. There may also be itching or a feeling of grittiness and a discharge or watering of the eye.

Antibiotics may be prescribed for a bacterial infection and antiallergy drugs for an allergic reaction. Conjunctivitis is self-limiting but infectious, so patients should use separate towels from the rest of their family. Bathing the eyes frequently in cooled boiled water may ease discomfort.

CORNEAL DYSTROPHY
A potentially sight-threatening condition in which dystrophy, or wasting, of the cornea causes it to lose transparency. Both eyes may be affected.

What are the causes?
There are 20 types of dystrophy, most of which are genetic. They are classified according to the area affected.
- **Epithelial dystrophies** The problem affects the outer layer of the cornea. An example is Cogan microcystic dystrophy.
- **Stromal dystrophies** The dystrophy affects the middle layer of the cornea, making it cloudy.
- **Endothelial dystrophies** The inside surface of the cornea is affected, as in the age-related Fuchs endothelial dystrophy.

What are the symptoms?
Many cases of Cogan dystrophy remain symptomless, although even in early stages telltale irregular patches can be spotted by an eye doctor. In some people, small areas of the outer layer of cells may break down, causing pain and watering. This may recur. Fuchs dystrophy is more common in women than in men, and sometimes a cataract is also present. It causes pain and irritation.

What are the treatment options?

There is no treatment for the underlying condition. Those affected receive support and advice on maximizing vision. The symptoms can be treated. Cell breakdown may be treated by patching the eye or with ointment; serious cases may need epithelial scraping to encourage new tissue growth. A corneal graft is an option in the most severe cases.

CORNEAL ULCER
A painful, inflammatory defect on the cornea.

What are the causes?

Corneal ulcers can result from infection, particularly with herpes virus. Contact lenses that have not been properly cleaned or stored or have been worn for longer than advised can also lead to infection and a corneal ulcer.

What are the symptoms?

Corneal ulcers give the feeling that there is a foreign body in the eye and can be painful. There may also be redness, watering, and sensitivity to light. Once the ulcer has healed, it may leave a scar.

How is it diagnosed?

During an eye examination, an ulcer will be visible as a white or gray indented spot on the corneal surface. The appearance of the ulcer under the slit lamp may give an indication of the infective organism, but the patient will need to be referred to an ophthalmologist for further investigation. Samples taken from the corneal surface will be cultured in the laboratory to identify the organism.

What are the treatment options?

Drugs can be used to help prevent the ulcer from spreading infection to other parts of the eye. Antibiotics or antivirals are used to treat any underlying infection. Any scar that is left after the ulcer heals will be permanent and, depending on its size and position, may interfere with vision.

CONTACT LENS COMPLICATIONS
Although most problems associated with contact lens wear are minor, a few will require treatment.

What are the causes?

Most contact lens problems arise from
• wearing contact lenses longer than advised,
• inadequate cleaning or disinfection of the lenses or storage case,
• using the wrong solutions,
• developing an allergic reaction to the lenses or solutions used to care for them.

Infections, allergies, dryness, swelling, and disruption of the corneal surface are possible complications of lens wear.

What are the symptoms?

Discomfort, redness, haziness of the cornea, and blurred vision can all indicate that something is wrong. If the symptoms persist or worsen once the lenses have been removed, the patient should seek urgent attention because some infections can progress rapidly.

If lenses are worn for longer than advised, the cornea's oxygen supply may be reduced, which may cause small blood vessels to grow into the cornea (neovascularization). This is the body's attempt to get more oxygen to the "starved" tissues. These vessels are fragile and can leak, causing visual loss. The problem is less acute if gas permeable lenses are worn.

In giant papillary conjunctivitis (GPC)—a complication associated with all types of lens—small, raised pustules occur inside the eyelid.

Some problems have no symptoms but can be picked up on examination by the optician. Contact lens wearers are, therefore, advised to have regular checkups.

How is it diagnosed?

During a routine eye examination, the optician puts a drop of an orange dye called fluorescein onto the eye and examines the surface with a slit lamp. Any scratches or breaks in the surface of the eye will fluoresce under the light of the microscope. The pattern of this fluorescence, as well as the appearance of the underside of the eyelid, provides the keys to diagnosis. Infections may require referral to an ophthalmologist, where samples can be taken from the ocular surface and cultured in the laboratory to identify the infectious agent.

What are the treatment options?

Careful attention to hygiene when handling lenses and strict adherence to instructions regarding lens care and storage will minimize the risk of developing a problem. Treatment of any complication depends on the underlying problem. For example, an allergic reaction will require a change in lens-care solutions; dryness can be treated by increasing blinking, changing to different lenses or using artificial tears. Sometimes patients are advised to wear lenses for a shorter time each day.

An allergy to a contact lens or solution may lead to a reaction such as that seen in allergic conjunctivitis or giant papillary conjunctivitis (GPC). Lenses should not be worn while the disease is active; when it has cleared, a new lens-cleaning solution can be tried. Infections are treated according to the microbe responsible (see Keratitis, p. 141).

DIABETIC RETINOPATHY
Damage to the retina caused by diabetes. The less well-controlled the diabetes and the longer the patient has been affected, the greater the effects of retinopathy.

What are the causes?
Diabetes affects all the small blood vessels of the body, including those of the eye, making them leaky. Blood and fluid leaking from these vessels solidify in the surrounding tissue. In severe cases, new, fragile vessels may grow into the area, and scar tissue forms, which can contract and cause retinal detachment (p. 143). The affected areas of the retina cannot detect light, so vision is impaired. The more central the damaged area, the worse the visual impairment.

What are the symptoms?
In the early stages of diabetic eye disease, there are no noticeable effects on vision. However, diabetics have regular eye examinations to monitor any changes in the retina.

How is it diagnosed?
The pupil is dilated and the inside of the eye is photographed to give an image of the blood vessels of the retina. An eye doctor may have a retinal camera that produces a computerized record of the appearance of the retina. This enables changes over time to be monitored.

What are the treatment options?
The better a patient's blood sugar levels are controlled, the less likely it is that severe sight problems will develop. Some of the leaky and fragile vessels can be closed using a laser, the mainstay of treatment. If laser treatment fails, new blood vessels and fibrous tissue will form. This can lead to retinal detachment and severe glaucoma can develop. Most diabetic eye care is shared among eye doctors, the family doctor, and other health professionals. About 2 percent of diabetics do lose their sight.

DRY EYES
Abnormal dryness of the usually moist eye surface.

What are the causes?
There are a number of possible causes of dryness, such as prominent eyes, reduced tear production, imbalance in the composition of the tears, menopause, reduced blinking (for example, during computer use), and working or living in a dry atmosphere. Dry eyes are also associated with certain diseases, such as the connective tissue disorder Sjögren's syndrome and certain types of arthritis, and are an occasional complication of drugs, including contraceptives.

What are the symptoms?
A dry, gritty, or burning irritation of the eye is common and it may feel as though a foreign body is present. Vision may be blurred. Vessels on the surface of the white of the eye may become prominent. Surprisingly, some people with dry eye problems notice that their eyes are watery—a reflex response to the irritation.

How is it diagnosed?
There are tests to determine whether the problem is a lack of tears or one of the components of tears, such as moisture or oils. In Schirmer's test, a strip of paper is inserted inside the lower lid to soak up the tears. How wet the paper is after a given period indicates whether levels of tear production are normal.

"Tear break-up time" indicates whether the mucin component of the tears is lacking. A drop of the orange dye fluorescein is put into the eye, and after a couple of blinks, the patient is asked to refrain from blinking. The optician observes the dye under light from a slit lamp to see how long it takes for a dry spot to appear on the surface.

What are the treatment options?
Most cases of dryness are not serious and can be treated with artificial tears and blinking exercises. If left untreated, however, they can progress to inflammation of the cornea and conjunctiva. In some cases, tiny plugs may be inserted to close the ducts through which the tears drain away, trapping the tears on the eyes' surface.

ECTROPION AND ENTROPION
Abnormal positions of the edge of the lower lid. In entropion the lid turns inward, in ectropion it turns out.

Entropion brings the lower lashes into contact with the eye, which can cause irritation. Ectropion moves the tear drainage ducts outward, so tears may run over the cheeks. Both conditions occur more frequently with increasing age. Either can be caused by shrinkage of scar tissue on the lid. Entropion can also be caused by shrinkage of the conjunctiva or the tissues that cushion the eyeball. Surgery can correct both conditions.

FLASHES AND FLOATERS
Also known as photopsia, flashes of light or color may appear in the vision. Floaters are small dark specks.

What are the causes?
Floaters are strands of condensed matter in the vitreous humor, the jelly that fills the back of the eyeball. Flashes may occur when pressure is applied to a closed eye; they can also arise from nerve damage. Gradual retinal damage—such as in diabetic eye disease—can cause tears or holes to form, which can lead to retinal detachment, as can injury.

What are the symptoms?
Floaters are rarely cause for concern. However, a large number of them, particularly in combination with flashes, requires urgent medical attention because they can indicate detachment of either the vitreous humor or a tear or detachment of the retina.

How is it diagnosed?
The report of flashes and floaters will prompt internal examination of the eye. An ophthalmoscope can give a view of only a limited portion of the retina; drops are needed to dilate the pupil and give a better viewing area. A physician or optician should refer the patient to an ophthalmologist, where an instrument that gives a complete view of the retina can be used.

What are the treatment options?
Detachment of the jelly filling the eye is not in itself harmful, although it can pull the retina away as it detaches (see Retinal detachment, p. 143).

GIANT CELL ARTERITIS
This condition is also called temporal arteritis when it affects the arteries in the temples.

What are the causes?
This is a disease in which the elastic tissue in the walls of arteries becomes inflamed, which can lead to narrowing and blockage of the arteries. It may affect arteries in other areas of the body, but the head and neck are generally first affected, which results in insufficient oxygen supply to the tissues in this area. The disease is most common in people in their 70s or 80s. Degeneration of the optic nerve occurs in about one in four patients with giant cell arteritis.

What are the symptoms?
Initially, patients may have a headache, scalp tenderness, and pain in the jaw. Muscle pain and weakness may also occur. The optic nerve problems associated with the condition arise quickly—within weeks of the condition appearing. Transient loss of vision and seeing flashing lights may precede a profound, irreversible loss of vision.

How is it diagnosed?
Inflammation is seen in the temporal arteries and, as the disease gets worse, it is no longer possible to feel a pulse here. A biopsy is taken from the arteries, and blood tests can confirm the diagnosis. It is not possible to predict which patients will develop optic nerve disease, and sight loss may have occurred in one eye by the time of diagnosis. It is often this that prompts a patient to seek treatment.

What are the treatment options?
This condition requires urgent medical attention. Steroid therapy should be started quickly (before the biopsy results) to prevent further optic nerve damage. In a patient with one affected eye, steroids may prevent damage to the unaffected eye.

GLAUCOMA
A group of sight-threatening conditions, usually involving pressure changes within the eye, which can cause irreversible damage to the optic nerve.

What are the causes?
There are three types of glaucoma:
- Congenital glaucoma is rare and inherited, and it occurs in babies and young children.
- Closed-angle glaucoma is a rapidly progressing condition that requires urgent treatment. There is also a chronic, slow-developing form more common in the Far East.
- Open-angle glaucoma, the third and most common form, is a progressive long-term condition, which rarely appears before the age of 40. It is rare in Caucasians.

Estimates suggest that about 93 million people worldwide have glaucoma, about one tenth of whom are blind in both eyes. Rates of blindness are lower in the developed world, where more people have access to health care.

In all three types, the drainage system for the fluid filling the front of the eye becomes blocked. This can cause a rapid increase in pressure inside the eye, which results in optic nerve damage and loss of vision. Closed-angle glaucoma is more common in people with hypermetropia (p. 140), some of whom have shallow anterior chambers. It can also result from other conditions, such as uveitis (p. 145).

Open-angle glaucoma is difficult to detect. It develops insidiously and sometimes can be the result of another condition, such as injury. It is more common in those with a family history of the disease, people of Afro-Caribbean origin, people with diabetes, and those with myopia (p. 142). There is normally—although not always—increased pressure within the eye. About one in seven of the people with this higher-than-normal pressure will develop glaucoma; the higher the pressure, the greater the risk. Large variation in pressure within the eye at different times of day is common in people with glaucoma.

What are the symptoms?
- Congenital glaucoma causes enlargement of the eyeball.
- Acute closed-angle glaucoma causes severe pain, a red circle around the edge of the iris, and blurred vision. The pupil is fixed, dilated, and often oval. Occasionally, the pressure buildup may be intermittent and few symptoms may arise.
- Open-angle glaucoma has no symptoms until the damage is severe, when there may be blurred vision, haloes seen around lights, and loss of peripheral vision—tunnel vision.

How is it diagnosed?
- In congenital glaucoma, the cornea is cloudy at birth and the eye becomes enlarged within 3 years.
- In closed-angle glaucoma, observation of the anterior chamber using a technique known as gonioscopy will reveal the narrowing of the anterior chamber angle that restricts aqueous flow.
- Open-angle glaucoma is complex to diagnose and involves at least three different tests, which often need to be repeated on a separate occasion to give conclusive results. Observation of the disk of the optic nerve head shows it to be increasingly pale. A tonometer fitted to a slit lamp

is used to measure the flexibility of the surface of the eye; from this, the pressure of the fluid inside the eye can be calculated. The final piece of the puzzle is a visual field test that measures any blind spots in the patient's vision (these will not be noticed by the patient until the very advanced stages of glaucoma).

What are the treatment options?
Surgery to improve aqueous drainage is the main treatment for congenital glaucoma.

For acute closed-angle glaucoma, medication is used to lower pressure in the eye before surgery. Peripheral iridectomy is the treatment of choice. This involves making a laser or surgical hole through the iris so that the iris can "flap back" into place, opening up the chamber angle.

In open-angle glaucoma, eye drops are used to lower the pressure inside the eye, which generally prevents further damage. If this fails, a trabulectomy is an option; this creates a bypass route for fluid to exit the eye.

HORDEOLUM (STY)
A pus-producing infection of a gland or lash follicle. On the outer surface of the lid, the condition is called an external hordeolum, commonly known as a sty. On the inner surface of the lid, it is called an internal hordeolum.

A sty occurs more often in people with blepharitis (p. 135) and in those with reduced resistance to infection. The usual infectious agent is a staphylococcus bacterium. A tender, swollen red lump develops quickly on the lid margin. Discomfort is greater with an internal hordeolum. Sties normally get better without treatment, although bathing the eye in previously boiled water can ease discomfort. An internal hordeolum may leave a small hard nodule after it bursts; this can be removed by minor surgery.

HYPERMETROPIA (HYPEROPIA)
Farsightedness—objects close to the eye are blurred and some people also have blurred distance vision.

What are the causes?
If the refractive system of the eye bends light from close objects too little, it will fail to bring the objects into focus before the light reaches the retina. Hypermetropia is usually inherited and is generally the result of an eyeball that is not long enough.

How is it diagnosed?

A patient is asked to keep his or her eyes fixed on a target in an autorefractor so that the machine can make an estimate of a prescription. Alternatively, the optician may use a retinoscope. By observing the movement of a beam of light shone through the pupil on to the retina, the optician can estimate the type and degree of refractive error.

These results are refined using a chart printed with different-sized letters, which the patient is asked to read with the help of lenses of different powers. The patient also looks at a target that is half red and half green.

What are the treatment options?

The problem is corrected with glasses or contact lenses. The lenses used have a convex surface that causes light rays to converge a little before they enter the eye. Refractive surgery is becoming an increasingly popular means of vision correction and is suitable for low hypermetropic prescriptions.

KERATITIS
Inflammation of the cornea.

What are the causes?

The most common cause of keratitis is infection by one or more bacteria, including pseudomonades, staphylococci, and streptococci. It may also be caused by viruses, fungi, or the Acanthamoeba amoeba. Occasionally keratitis appears in the skin condition rosacea, which causes persistent facial redness, frequent flushing, and, sometimes, acne. Rosacea keratitis often arises between the ages of 30 and 50.

What are the symptoms?

Pain, redness, and blurred vision are common. The pain may take the form of an aching sensation.

How is it diagnosed?

The cornea is examined closely because a variety of corneal changes may be seen in different forms of keratitis. If infection is suspected, samples are taken from the surface or a biopsy of corneal tissue may be taken if the infection is in the lower layer of the cornea. Organisms from these samples are grown in the laboratory to aid identification.

What are the treatment options?

Some eye infections progress rapidly, so a broad-spectrum antibiotic will be given immediately. When the particular infectious organism is identified, antiviral, antifungal, or antiamebic agents may be applied as drops or ointments. Once the condition has healed, permanent scars may remain. If these are extensive and interfere with vision, a corneal transplant may be required. In rosacea, keratitis is treated with short-term steroid drops.

KERATOCONUS
A progressive bulging of the cornea that usually first appears in the teenage years.

What are the causes?

Keratoconus runs in families. It is more common in those who suffer from allergies such as eczema and in people with Down's or Turner's syndrome.

What are the symptoms?

Vision is blurred and progressively deteriorates, which means that frequent changes of eyeglass prescription are needed.

How is it diagnosed?

The standard sight test by an optician will show increasing amounts of irregular astigmatism (p. 134) and myopia (p. 142), which eventually become difficult to correct with contact lenses. A technique called keratometry is used to plot the shape of the cornea, which shows a distinctive cone shape. Examination of the eye using a slit lamp shows fine, deep lines in the cornea. When the patient looks down, the lower lid bulges because of the bulging cornea.

What are the treatment options?

Rigid contact lenses are helpful in the early stages of the condition, but they do not halt the changes. Although progression may stop without treatment, in severe cases a corneal transplant is needed. This is usually very successful.

MACULAR HOLE
A hole in the macula, the part of the retina where the best daylight vision occurs.

Contraction of the jelly filling the back of the eye pulls the retina away from the underlying layers at the macula. A difference may be noticed in central vision when one eye is closed (for example, an object the patient is looking at may disappear). Blurred vision may be noticed. The condition is more common in older women, and sometimes both eyes are affected.

Examination of the retina with an ophthalmoscope will show an area of detachment at the macula. An eye specialist may use an imaging technique called fluorescein angiography to confirm the diagnosis. Surgery is sometimes effective at closing the hole, and vision may improve somewhat. Patients may also learn to cope with the condition by looking at objects slightly off-center.

MELANOMA
A malignant tumor of pigment cells. About 80 percent of melanomas of the eye occur in the choroid.

What are the symptoms?
The development of malignant tumors is a complex process with many contributing factors. There are often no symptoms, but vision may be blurred in some cases. About one in three patients complain of balls of light traveling across his or her vision (larger than the tiny flashes experienced with other conditions; see p. 139).

How is it diagnosed?
A routine eye examination will usually pick up signs of a tumor, even though a small tumor may be symptomless. The optician will refer the patient to an ophthalmologist.

Choroidal melanoma is a rare type of cancer, but it is the most common form of eye cancer.

Examination of the eye using a binocular indirect ophthalmoscope will show a brownish mass and often fluid under the retina, which can cause detachment as well as subtle changes in the retina. Ultrasound scans confirm the diagnosis.

What are the treatment options?
The treatment will depend on the size and position of the tumor; combinations of radiation and laser therapy are common. Removal of the eye may be necessary if the tumor is large. Melanoma can spread to other tissues of the body if not treated early, and the prognosis is not good if this has already occurred at the time of detection.

MYOPIA
Nearsightedness—objects in the distance are blurred, and patients sometimes experience headaches.

What are the causes?
The refractive system of the eye bends light from a distant object too much, bringing it in focus in front of rather than on the retina. It is usually the result of a slightly elongated eyeball and is generally inherited.

A progressive and severe form of myopia called high myopia (prescription of at least –6.00 D) can develop in late childhood and continue to worsen throughout adult life. It is associated with an increased risk of degenerative changes in the lens, retina, and choroid during young adulthood, but not all people with prescriptions of –6.00 D or more have the progressive condition. Those with high myopia are at increased risk of developing macular holes, retinal detachment, cataract, and open-angle glaucoma.

How is it diagnosed?
As with diagnosing hypermetropia (p. 140), the optician gains an initial estimate of the patient's prescription using an autorefractor or a retinoscope and then refines the estimate by noting the patient's reaction to printed letters when viewed through combinations of lenses of different power. Progressive high myopia is diagnosed when the degree of myopia does not stabilize but continues to increase.

What are the treatment options?
Glasses or contact lenses will be prescribed. The lens required has a concave surface that causes light rays to diverge a little before entering the eye. Refractive surgery is an increasingly popular treatment for low to moderate myopia, although it is unsuitable for high prescriptions. In high myopia, vision is commonly not fully corrected by glasses and, because of the risk of other sight-threatening conditions, patients are carefully monitored.

OCCLUSION, RETINAL VEIN/ARTERY
Blockage of the blood vessels of the retina that may cause permanent loss of vision.

What are the causes?
Raised blood pressure, diabetes, and hypermetropia (p. 140) increase the risk of retinal vein occlusion. Most of those affected are in their 60s or 70s. Retinal artery occlusion may occur as a result of heart disease, vascular disease, or the immune system disorder lupus. Retinal occlusion is more common in smokers. Arterial occlusion has a more severe effect on vision.

What are the symptoms?
The patient suddenly experiences partial loss of vision in one eye but no pain. Vision loss is complete if the main

artery is blocked. In vein occlusion, the vision is often said to be like "looking through smoke."

How is it diagnosed?
Examination will determine the type and severity of loss of vision. The appearance of the retina and blood vessels through an ophthalmoscope enable an initial diagnosis to be made, which is then confirmed by examining the blood flow through the retina using fluorescein angiography. The pupil of an affected retina is unresponsive to bright light.

What are the treatment options?
Urgent treatment is needed when the main artery is affected because the blockage starves the retina of oxygen. If the blockage is successfully removed within a day or so, vision may recover. Treatment involves reducing the pressure inside the eye using drugs and applying pressure to dislodge the blockage. Unfortunately, treatment is often unsuccessful.

Only a few vein occlusion cases cause the retina to become starved of oxygen, and after a few months, unaffected vessels may increase their capacity; blood flow may return to near normal and vision may recover. Even so, problems can persist. A small daily dose of aspirin may reduce the chances of further occlusive episodes.

OPTIC NEURITIS
Inflammation of the optic nerve.

What are the causes?
Three times more women than men are affected by optic neuritis, which is a loss of the myelin covering around the nerve fibers so that they cannot function properly.

What are the symptoms?
Central vision declines over several days. There may be pain when moving the affected eye and a frontal headache.

How is it diagnosed?
A letter test chart measures the amount of vision loss. A visual field test, in which the patient looks at a central target while tiny lights flash around the edges of the viewing area, is also conducted. Optic neuritis makes the patient less able to see the lights in the center than those toward the edges of their vision. There are also problems with the pupil's response to light, with color vision and with loss of contrast sensitivity.

Optic neuritis most commonly occurs during the 20s, but it can happen at any time. In 70 percent of cases, only one eye is involved.

What are the treatment options?
Vision often returns to normal within about a month, although it may take longer, but the inability to see clearly in low-contrast conditions may persist. Drugs may help reduce the severity of an attack. In some patients, the diagnosis of optic neuritis is the first sign of more serious neurological problems, such as multiple sclerosis.

PAPILLEDEMA
A swelling of the head of the optic nerve as a result of raised pressure of the fluid in the brain.

What are the causes?
Elevated pressure in the fluid of the brain leading to this condition can be brought on by head injury, brain or optic nerve tumor, bleeding into the space between the membranes of the brain, high blood pressure, or encephalitis.

What are the symptoms?
Severe headaches are common. The first eye symptoms may be transient loss of vision in one or both eyes—for example, when the person stands up. Vision may gradually worsen. The field of view may become narrow.

How is it diagnosed?
The optic nerve is a visible part of the central nervous system and gives valuable early warning of problems in the brain. Early signs of changes in the disk of the optic nerve head can be picked up using an ophthalmoscope. The disk looks red and swollen, and the small blood vessels that cross it are difficult to see. There are subtle changes in the appearance of the nerve at different stages of the disease. The patient may be referred to the hospital for tests.

What are the treatment options?
Effective treatment of the underlying condition can prevent further damage to the optic nerve. Treatment will depend on the problem within the central nervous system.

RETINAL BREAK
Retinal breaks are divided into retinal tears and retinal holes depending on shape, size, nature, and distribution. Tears may be horseshoe-shaped; holes are round.

As we age, the edge of the vitreous humour pulls away from the retina, a process called posterior vitreous detachment (PVD). For most people this causes no problem, but in some the vitreous humor "tugs" on the retina to produce a break. The area affected is unable to function. The more central and extensive the damage, the more it may threaten vision. If fluid seeps into the break, it can produce a retinal detachment.

RETINAL DETACHMENT
A separation of the part of the retina containing the nerves from the pigment layer at the point where light receptors meet the retinal pigment layer. This is a sight-threatening condition that needs urgent treatment.

What are the causes?
Retinal detachment occurs most commonly in the nearsighted, those with a family history of the condition, and those who have had cataract surgery, an inflammation of the eye, or an eye injury. There are three main types:
- In a simple detachment, liquid from the vitreous enters breaks in the retina and opens them up, separating the light receptors from the retina.
- A second type is associated with inflammation in which the fluid causing the detachment is leakage from the inflamed vessels of the choroid.
- If a repair of a simple detachment fails, a complex detachment, in which scar tissue pulls the retina away from its supporting tissue, may occur. This is relatively rare.

What are the symptoms?
A patient may notice flashes and floaters, a sign that a retinal break may have occurred, and go to the eye hospital because of the risk of a detachment. There is a rapid deterioration in vision—over days rather than weeks.

How is it diagnosed?
The diagnosis is made on the basis of the reported symptoms and an examination of the retina.

What are the treatment options?
For simple detachments, a gas bubble is injected into the eye to put pressure on the retina and move it back into place. After a couple of weeks, laser or crythotherapy is used to seal the retina in place. Some detachments are best treated with a silicone band, which is attached to the outside of the eye to press the retina back into place. This band is not visible and stays in place. Again, laser or cryotherapy may be useful. See page 105.

RETINITIS PIGMENTOSA
A group of progressive, sight-threatening conditions in which the retina degenerates.

What are the causes?
The conditions are inherited and differ in age of onset and severity. The rod cells responsible for vision in low-light conditions and the pigment layer of the retina are affected. Pigment accumulates in parts of the retina, interfering with cell function; blood supply is reduced; and eventually there is wasting of the optic nerve.

What are the symptoms?
The first symptom is night blindness. The visual field becomes restricted, but this is not usually noticed until the condition is advanced. By the age of 50, many sufferers have poor vision, and most will lose nearly all of their sight.

How is it diagnosed?
A detailed family history is necessary. A visual field test shows progressive reduction of the field of vision, and the retina shows distinctive changes as dark blobs of pigment accumulate. Electrical recordings of eye movement and of the sensitivity of the retina to light will be made.

What are the treatment options?
No treatment can halt the progression of the condition, but low-vision aids can help with daily activities.

SCLERITIS
A rare but potentially serious condition affecting the white of the eye, the sclera.

In scleritis, severe inflammation can cause the sclera to waste away, with the result that an eye can be lost. Early diagnosis is not easy, especially if the condition develops at the back of the sclera, which is difficult to see even on detailed examination. The condition is extremely painful and can cause the sclera to have a bluish appearance. Treatment is with high doses of steroids or other immunosuppressive drugs.

Inflammation of the superficial layers of the sclera, usually referred to as episcleritis, is mild and self-limiting, and generally does not require any treatment.

SQUINT (STRABISMUS)
A condition in which one eye fails to point at the object being viewed. Esotropia is movement of the eye toward the nose; movement away from the nose is exotropia.

.

What are the causes?
Squint in childhood is caused by a failure of the signaling pathways between eye and brain. In adults, it results from problems in the extraocular muscles that control eye movement. Childhood squints often run in families.

What are the symptoms?
The eyes do not move in a coordinated way when a person looks in a particular direction; sometimes the problem is only apparent when one eye is covered. A person may also alter the resting position of the head to compensate for an eye that does not have the full range of movement and may experience double vision. An uncorrected childhoood squint can lead to amblyopia (p. 134).

How is it diagnosed?
Tests for stereovision will be conducted and the movement of each eye observed with the other eye covered and uncovered. The inside of the eye is examined (with drops to dilate the pupil) to look for any underlying eye disease.

What are the treatment options?
Glasses may be prescribed. Amblyopia therapy (covering one eye with a patch) may also be tried. An orthoptist may prescribe a series of eye exercises. If these methods are unsuccessful, surgery may be necessary to bring the squinting eye back into alignment and establish binocular vision.

TRACHOMA
Sight-threatening infection of the conjunctiv, spread by poor hygiene. It is more common, but less serious, in children than in adults.

Infection with chlamydia is responsible for this condition, which often occurs in children and is the most common preventable cause of blindness, particularly in developing countries. Dry eye and conjunctivitis progress, if untreated, to produce severe scarring of the conjunctiva, eyelid deformity, and, eventually, corneal ulcers. The condition can be treated with oral antibiotics, primarily tetracyline ointment, although once severe problems have developed, damage cannot be reversed. Children tend to recover, although reinfection is common. Poor access to medical care means that many adults lose their sight.

Six million people worldwide have been blinded by trachoma; 600 million people are at risk worldwide.

UVEITIS
Anterior uveitis (also referred to as iritis) is inflammation of the iris and the ciliary body; posterior uveitis is inflammation of the choroid.

What are the causes?
Both forms may be local or part of a systemic inflammatory disease. Trauma is a common cause of local uveitis. Systemic causes of anterior uveitis include ankylosing spondilitis, gastrointestinal inflammation, juvenile arthritis, and sarcoidosis. Sarcoidosis is also a potential cause of posterior uveitis, but the most common cause in the developed world is toxoplasmosis, spread by an organism whose main host is the domestic cat.

What are the symptoms?
The symptoms vary according to the speed of development and the part of the uvea most affected. Iritis, which develops rapidly, produces a painful, red, watery eye; sensitivity to light; and floaters (p. 139), caused by cells leaking into the fluid in front of the lens. Vision may be blurred or hazy and the pupil constricted. There are fewer symptoms when the choroid is affected—primarily floaters.

How is it diagnosed?
Eye examination with a slit lamp will show signs of cell and other debris in the fluid contents of the eye, as well as the iris sticking to the lens or cornea. There may be deposits in the cornea. Pupil responses to light are affected. Examination of the choroid and retina can also provide information to help identify the problem.

What are the treatment options?
Active iritis is treated with steroid drops or ointment, or in severe cases, steroid injections. Oral steroids can suppress the inflammation in posterior uveitis, but if toxoplasmosis is a factor, antimicrobial drugs are also needed.

THE MOUTH

ABSCESS
A localized collection of dead tissue, fluid, bacteria, and living and dead white blood cells.

What are the causes?
Dental abscesses are caused by pus-forming bacteria. If the bacteria multiply, the abscess can enlarge and some of the pus-filled cells are replaced by scar tissue.

What are the symptoms?
There are two types of dental abscess:
- A peri-apical abscess forms in the bone on the end of the root of a tooth when infection and pus spread from tooth pulp that has "died" as a result of caries (p. 147). The caries may have caused a throbbing toothache.
- A periodontal abscess forms in the gum at the side of the root as a consequence of periodontal disease. It will be painful, but the pain may resolve if the abscess bursts.

How is it diagnosed?
A tooth with a periodontal abscess will be painful when given a gentle tap by the dentist. There will be pus draining from a sinus or directly from a swelling on the gum next to the affected tooth. A tooth with a peri-apical abscess will not respond to heat, cold, or electrical stimuli.

What are the treatment options?
Any abscess needs to be drained of pus and may need to be incised. A tooth with a peri-apical abscess will require root canal therapy or extraction. A tooth with a periodontal abscess will need thorough cleaning of calculus, plaque and debris from below the gum line. If the tooth is badly affected, extraction may be necessary.

APHTHOUS ULCER
A common condition affecting one fifth of the population.

What are the causes?
In the majority of cases, the cause of an ulcer in unknown. Sometimes a deficiency of iron, vitamin B_{12}, or folic acid may be responsible; other causes are injury and stress.

What are the symptoms?
The main symptom is a sharp, needlelike pain at the affected site, which may become so acute that eating and talking are difficult. The symptoms may stem from a single lesion or from multiple ulcers around the mouth. The painful affected areas are usually on the sides of the tongue or inside the lips and cheeks.

How is it diagnosed?
The pale appearance and soreness and pain are characteristic, although a blood test may be indicated to check for vitamin deficiency. Recurrence of ulcers every 3 to 6 months or more frequently confirms the diagnosis.

What are the treatment options?
Ulcers will heal after 10 to 14 days without any treatment; over-the-counter gels and creams will relieve discomfort. Topical steroid creams or pellets may help in severe cases. Any dental problems that might have triggered the ulcer(s) should be resolved. If nutritional deficiencies are detected, vitamin B_{12} and folic acid supplements will be given. An antibacterial mouthwash may help prevent infection of the ulcers.

BRUXISM
A common condition affecting both children and adults.

Bruxism is the habit of grinding or clenching the teeth while sleeping, although it may also persist during waking hours. If unrecognized or untreated, the chronic effects of bruxism on the dental and oral tissues can be difficult to treat.

What are the causes?
The habit may be precipitated by a simple, local cause such as a high spot on a filling or an erupting tooth; the jaws are clenched to try to find a comfortable biting position. Stress is another cause because the subconscious habit of grinding the teeth is one means through which tension may be eased.

What are the symptoms?
The person involved may not be aware of any symptoms, but a sleeping partner may hear the sound of forceful tooth grinding. It is, however, more common for symptoms associated with bruxism, such as pain in the jaw joints and progressive wearing away of the teeth, to be reported.

What are the treatment options?
Any local dental factors that might be triggering the habit should be treated and underlying lifestyle stresses identified. If required, the patient should be referred to a doctor for

further assessment. A plastic splint that fits over the teeth and is worn during sleep may prevent the habit and protect tooth surfaces from further wear.

BURNING MOUTH
A disorder predominantly affecting females.

Burning mouth may be a sign of a nondental condition and, rarely, a symptom of a serious disorder.

What are the causes?
It is not always possible to identify one specific cause. Underlying anemia may be influential, precipitated by a deficiency of iron or vitamin B_{12}; diabetes, or factors such as stress or depression. Possible dental causes include an allergy to the metal or plastic components of a denture or a filling. Food allergies or a reaction to a toothpaste, as well as dentures that don't fit properly or are too bulky, are also common triggers.

What are the symptoms?
The burning or itching can start in the morning and increase in severity, becoming painful. The tongue is most commonly affected, but there are rarely obvious signs of the problem for the dentist to see. A patient may complain of a dry mouth.

What are the treatment options?
A suspected underlying disorder such as diabetes or a dietary deficiency should be treated. A doctor can help with management of stress, anxiety, or depression. A dentist can remake poorly fitting dentures and treat any dental disease. When an allergy is confirmed by patch testing, the offending material needs to be eliminated.

CANCER
One of the most serious disorders affecting the mouth.

Cancer can affect almost any part of the mouth, including the tongue, mouth floor, lips, gums, inside of the cheeks, palate, sinuses, and salivary glands.

What are the symptoms?
Oral cancer is likely to appear as an ulcer, but it may not be painful until a late stage. Any ulcer that persists longer than 2 to 3 weeks should be checked by a dentist. If the ulcerated area becomes infected, a bad taste can develop.

What are the causes?
For cancers of the floor of mouth, tongue, and lips, smoking and alcohol are major risk factors, especially if combined. Pipe smoking and prolonged exposure to sunlight have been implicated in lip cancer. Chronic, long-term irritation and injury from sharp teeth or fillings may also be important.

What are the treatment options?
Surgical excision and radiation, often in combination, are the treatments of choice. When surgery involves the jaws or face, reconstructive surgery may be recommended.

What is the outlook?
Early diagnosis and treatment are crucial. There is a major risk that long-standing lesions, particularly those of the tongue and floor of the mouth, may spread to the head, neck, and lymph nodes. The prognosis is considerably less optimistic when the cancer has spread.

CARIES
One of the most widespread diseases in the West, caries has been reducing in incidence in recent years.

All parts of a tooth are at risk from dental caries, which first affects the surface enamel and spreads to the dentin. When cavities have been filled, caries can develop at the margins between the filling and the tooth or underneath the filling. The exposed roots of teeth are also at risk.

Most developed countries and many nonindustrial nations have now reached the World Health Organization goal of individuals under the age of 12 having fewer than three decayed, missing, or filled teeth.

What are the causes?
Caries is the result of loss of mineral in the form of calcium and phosphate ions from the tooth surface, caused mainly by species of bacteria that metabolize sugar into acid. Other significant factors are the the frequency of eating or snacking (including taking sugar in tea or coffee), the amount of sugar in the diet, having an adequate flow of saliva, and the resistance of the tooth to caries.

What are the symptoms?
Symptoms only appear late in the process, when the caries has affected the dentin and possibly also the pulp of the tooth. When the pulp is involved (see Pulpitis, p. 153), toothache will be experienced. With advanced, gross caries, the main part of the tooth decays and is unsightly.

How is it diagnosed?

The dentist uses a mirror with good illumination to identify the presence of caries. A fine, sharp dental probe is used to feel for caries that may be progressing at sites that are difficult to see. X rays will show caries at various stages of progression, although the decay may be slightly more advanced on the tooth than it appears on an X ray.

The number of adults ages 18 to 34 missing all their natural teeth has declined from 2 percent in the early 1980s to 0.4 percent.

What are the treatment options?

Provided that the surface of the tooth has not completely broken down, an attempt can be made to remineralize the surface through dietary changes and the use of fluoride. Otherwise, treatment involves drilling out the caries and filling the tooth or, in some cases, removing the tooth.

CLEFT LIP AND PALATE
A cleft is a split in the lip or palate or both on one (unilateral) or both (bilateral) sides of the mouth.

Both conditions range from slight to severe: Cleft lips range from minor "nicks" to gaps from lip to nose and occasionally into the nose; a cleft palate may be a small space in the soft palate or an almost complete separation in the roof of the mouth extending into the nasal cavity. The gums may also be affected.

What are the causes?

Clefts occur when parts of the facial anatomy of a fetus that should fuse together during pregnancy fail to do so. It is unclear why this happens. The likelihood of a cleft is higher if another member of the family has one, but they also often occur where there is no previous history.

How is it diagnosed?

A diagnosis can often be made from an ultrasound scan; otherwise, the problem is obvious from the appearance. Babies with a cleft palate may also have difficulty feeding. Depending on the extent of the cleft, feeding using specially designed bottles and nipples may be helpful.

What are the treatment options?

A cleft lip will be repaired when a baby is about 3 months old. A palate is usually repaired later, at about a year old. Several operations may be necessary as the child grows.

What is the outlook?

Speech development will be monitored, although children with a cleft lip or gum usually speak well. Palate patients may require speech therapy. Middle ear infections tend to be more common in children with a cleft palate and ear tubes may be needed to improve hearing. Tooth development may also be affected, with orthodontic treatment needed when the permanent teeth come through.

COLD SORE
A cold sore is a sign of a recurring viral infection.

A cold sore, also known as herpes labialis, is seen most commonly as a small, irregular, reddened area at the border between the lip and the skin of the face. After a primary infection (see Herpes infection, p. 151), the virus remains dormant in the central part of one of the nerves that relay sensory information from the face and mouth to the brain. A number of factors, including sunlight, stress, or being generally unwell, can then reactivate this "sleeping" virus.

The initial symptom is a tingling or itchy sensation felt at the area of the lip where the cold sore is developing. A blister forms and loses its top to leave an open sore. These sores are recurrent, so most individuals recognize the problem quickly. An antiviral cream can be applied to the sore regularly for about a week or until the lesion heals. Treatment should be started as soon as the tingling is felt.

CYSTS
A cyst is a cavity lined with epithelium that contains a fluid or a semisolid material.

There are many types of cysts that form in and around the jaws; the most common are associated with the teeth.

What are the causes?

The formation of a cyst is linked to a structure that develops entirely or in part from epithelium. The tooth enamel is derived from epithelium, and consequently there are islands of epithelial tissue in the bones of the jaw that can begin to grow. Some of the developing epithelium degenerates to form the fluid content of the cyst, and a layer of cells remains as the lining. A cyst may be associated with a tooth or it may replace the tooth in its entirety. Cysts may also develop in the inflammatory tissue of long-standing abscesses on the sides or at the ends of the roots of a tooth.

What are the symptoms?

Many cysts are completely symptom-free. When a cyst develops from an old abscess, the tooth will usually have been painful in the past. A cyst on the gums or associated with erupting teeth may be recognized as a bluish swelling below the gum surface. Some cysts form in the bone; if undiagnosed and not treated, they may grow to such an extent that the jaw expands and adjacent teeth may be displaced.

What are the treatment options?

Cysts can be removed surgically, although there is a danger that the lining may rupture, making recurrence a problem. Very large cysts can be opened and made continuous with the mouth; over time, the cyst space will fill with new bone. Teeth with chronic abscesses that have developed into cysts require root canal therapy.

DENTURE-INDUCED STOMATITIS

A fungal infection that can be associated with wearing dentures.

What are the causes?

Denture-induced stomatitis is caused, at least in part, by the fungus *Candida albicans,* which is present in most people's mouths. The problem is more likely to develop when dentures are old or are rarely removed.

What are the symptoms?

The area beneath the denture becomes red and sore and may lead to the complaint of a "burning" sensation. These symptoms are almost always associated with an upper denture. Soreness at the corners of the mouth is typical of a condition called angular cheilitis, which is also caused by the fungus and may be present in people who wear dentures.

How is it diagnosed?

A dentist will recognize the characteristic redness and swelling of the gums and palate: The redness matches almost exactly the outline of the denture. A culture taken from the tissues or from the denture will confirm the presence of the fungus if there is any doubt of the diagnosis.

What are the treatment options?

The dentures must be removed, cleaned thoroughly and regularly, and stored overnight in sterilizing solution. Any obvious defect of the dentures should be corrected. An antifungal cream can be applied to the affected tissues.

DRY SOCKET

Dry socket is the term used to describe a painful socket from which a tooth recently has been extracted.

This complication of tooth extraction occurs in less than 5 percent of cases. It is most common after a difficult extraction of a lower tooth at the back of the jaw. It seems to be more common in smokers than in nonsmokers.

What are the causes?

When a tooth is extracted, the socket usually fills up with blood to form a clot. If this clot fails to form properly or breaks up and is lost from the socket, it exposes the bone, and a dry socket is a likely consequence. It may become infected, although infection is not the cause of a dry socket.

What are the symptoms?

The extraction socket is extremely painful. This pain may not start immediately after the anesthetic injection wears off but often is delayed for 24 hours or even longer. There is usually also a bad taste in the mouth.

How is it diagnosed?

A dental inspection of the socket will reveal a "dry-looking" appearance to the bone that is exposed because of the lack of a blood clot. Small fragments or spikes of loose bone may also be seen in the socket.

What are the treatment options?

The dentist should clean any debris from the socket. The socket can then be washed and, if necessary, dressed using gauze and a preparation based on the chemical eugenol, such as oil of cloves. The dressing must be removed after a few days to allow healing to take place.

EPULIS

An epulis is a harmless localized swelling on the gum.

These lesions appear as small pink or red swellings that seem to be growing from the gum between teeth, usually toward the front of the mouth. Occasionally, they can grow large enough to cover the surface of a tooth.

What are the causes?

Irritation or injury to the gum by something as innocuous as a toothbrush bristle or an area of tartar on the teeth may cause chronic inflammation and trigger the growth of an epulis. The epulis forms over time as the gum tissue attempts to repair the damage and inflammation. An epulis may also calcify. They are fairly common during pregnancy.

What are the symptoms?

An epulis is not painful unless it grows to such a size that it interferes with eating. The constant friction from biting may lead to an ulcer on the surface. If the epulis contains a rich blood supply, it may bleed, either spontaneously or on brushing the associated teeth.

How is it diagnosed?

Diagnosis is by appearance. An X ray may be taken because, very occasionally, an epulis may be mistaken for another lesion that develops from within the bone of the jaw.

What are the treatment options?

An epulis is removed under local anesthesia. It can be difficult to ensure that all of the epulis has been removed, and recurrence is quite common.

GINGIVITIS
A common condition affecting both children and adults.

There are two forms of gingivitis: chronic gingivitis and acute necrotizing gingivitis, which is less common and appears like an acute infection. Acute gingivitis is more common in young adults and in the immunosuppressed.

What are the causes?

Chronic gingivitis is caused by a buildup of plaque, usually as a result of ineffective tooth brushing. Factors such as large fillings, crowns, dentures, and orthodontic braces may make brushing more difficult and indirectly lead to gingivitis.

Acute gingivitis may be caused by a specific bacterial infection. It is also linked to smoking and stress.

What are the symptoms?

Chronic gingivitis is only rarely painful, but the gums may be sore and bleed when the teeth are brushed. Bleeding can be spontaneous in more severe cases. Acute gingivitis is painful and may cause to a bad taste in the mouth and bad breath. The gums will bleed when the teeth are brushed.

How is it diagnosed?

Diagnosis is by the clinical appearance and symptoms. Chronic gingivitis is characterized by red, swollen gums that usually bleed when touched by a dental probe. In acute gingivitis, there are areas of ulceration on the gums. In severe cases, there is a characteristic foul smell.

What are the treatment options?

Both conditions are treated by improving the standard of oral hygiene and care. Calculus must be removed, and any factors that predispose to the buildup of plaque should be modified to make brushing easier. In acute gingivitis, an antibacterial mouthwash will clear debris and bacteria and antibiotics will speed recovery. Gingivitis is reversible, but if left untreated, it may progress to periodontitis (p. 152).

GINGIVAL ENLARGEMENT
Gingival enlargement is an overgrowth of the gums that can affect part or all of the mouth.

Gingival enlargement occurs most commonly when chronic gingivitis is long-standing and the body attempts to repair the damage caused by the inflammation.

Some drugs also cause enlargement of the gums. The main drugs involved are nifedipine, which reduces blood pressure; cyclosporine, which suppresses the immune system in people who have had organ transplants; and phenytoin, which is taken to control epileptic seizures. These drugs cause enlargement in 30 to 50 percent of cases, and the likelihood appears to be greater if oral hygiene is poor.

In severe cases that affect the gums at the front of the mouth, the main symptom is the appearance. The ability to chew may also be affected. Improvements in personal oral hygiene are vital, and then surgery can reduce the bulk of the overgrown tissue. Recurrence is possible, particularly when drugs cause the disorder; in these cases, the dentist may ask the physician if it is possible to prescribe an alternative drug without this side effect.

GINGIVAL RECESSION
Receding, or shrinkage, of the gums leading to the appearance of being "long in the tooth."

Gingival recession may occur around several teeth or adjacent to just one tooth, usually an incisor in the lower jaw. The well-known phrase "long in the tooth" implies that gum recession and exposure of the roots of the teeth is a consequence of the aging process. This is not strictly true, because many people are able to keep both their teeth and gums in excellent condition well into old age. Conversely, localized gingival recession often affects children and young adults.

What are the causes?

Gingival recession may be a consequence of periodontal disease—the gum tissue recedes when the bone supporting the teeth dissolves. The gums may also recede during or after orthodontic treatment. Perhaps the most common cause of recession, however, is injury, either from a habit such as chewing a pencil or from overenthusiastic tooth brushing.

When a tooth is out of line with the others in the jaw, the root may have only thin covering layers of bone and tissue. This will put the tooth at a higher risk of gum recession.

What are the symptoms?

At the front of the mouth, appearance may be a problem, although the lip almost always hides the area of gum recession. The exposed root of the tooth may be sensitive to touch, to hot and cold drinks, or even to cold air.

What are the treatment options?

The area of the recession must be kept as clean as possible by tooth brushing and polishing by the dentist. The dentist can also apply a varnish containing fluoride to harden the exposed root surface and make it less susceptible to caries in the long term. This varnish will also help if the tooth is sensitive to hot and cold temperatures.

In some cases, it may be possible to use a gum graft to cover part of the root of the tooth.

HALITOSIS

The term is derived from the Latin word halitus *and means foul or bad-smelling breath.*

Patients may confuse bad breath, which is halitosis, with a bad taste in the mouth. Frequently, when a patient complains of halitosis, bad breath cannot be detected by anyone else. In such cases, it is important to reassure the individual, because the perception that something is wrong for which no cause can be identified may lead to or be a symptom of depression.

What are the causes?

The bacteria that cause periodontal disease (p. 152) and gingivitis may lead to bad breath. The most well-known cause is acute gingivitis (p. 150). Viral infections of the mouth, throat, or any part of the upper gastrointestinal tract may also cause the problem. Smokers are at particular risk, and those who suffer from dry mouth (Xerostomia, p. 155) may also complain of a bad taste or bad breath.

How is it diagnosed?

It is necessary to establish whether the patient is suffering from a bad taste in the mouth or from bad breath. Decaying food debris stuck between teeth at a site that is difficult to clean frequently causes a bad taste rather than halitosis. Colonization by bacteria or plaque stagnation can cause similar problems.

Talking dries the mouth, making it friendly for the bacteria that cause halitosis, so those with jobs involving a lot of talking—teachers, lawyers, telemarketers— are at risk.

What are the treatment options?

Once the cause has been identified, the patient must be reassured that most cases are easily dealt with. Tooth brushing techniques should be improved and dental floss used where cleaning between the teeth is difficult. A mouth rinse can be used in the short term.

HERPES INFECTION

Infection with the herpes simplex 1 virus may be non-symptomatic or can give rise to an acute, debilitating condition seen mainly in young children.

The most common oral infection with herpes virus is herpetic gingivostomatitis. A baby gains temporary immunity from the infection through antibodies received from its mother—most adults have antibodies in their bloodstream, showing that they have acquired the virus at some time. After an infection, the virus remains dormant in the body and may be reactivated to produce a cold sore (p. 148).

In herpetic gingivostomatitis, the mouth becomes sore and eating difficult. The infection causes fever, high temperature, difficulty in swallowing, and enlarged lymph glands in the mouth and neck. Characteristic signs of the infection include red and inflamed gums and small fluid-filled blisters on the tongue, lips, and occasionally the palate. These burst to become small, round ulcers. A culture of a blister may be taken to confirm the presence of the virus.

The infection will resolve after 10 to 14 days, so treatment is directed toward making the child comfortable. Provide drinks to maintain fluid levels and a soft diet. Use damp gauze to clean the teeth if brushing is not possible. Liquid acetaminophen helps reduce fever.

LICHEN PLANUS
A condition seen mostly in middle-aged women in which lesions affect the skin as well as the mouth.

What are the causes?
The exact cause is not known, although anxiety, smoking, and diabetes have all been suggested. Trauma is an aggravating factor for lesions on the skin. Dental amalgam and some drugs, such as propanolol, may cause to lichen planus–like lesions in the mouth, so-called lichenoid reactions.

What are the symptoms?
Lichen planus may appear in a number of ways in the mouth. Classically, the insides of the cheeks have a covering of interweaving white streaks on the surface, and the tongue and gums may be affected. Occasionally, the lesions may be more extensive and be interspersed with inflamed red areas. Ulceration may occur, causing soreness and pain of varying severity. Symptoms may also be mild.

How is it diagnosed?
Visual inspection of the lesions is usually all that is needed for a diagnosis to be made. When there is some doubt, a biopsy will confirm the suspicion.

What are the treatment options?
No treatment other than reassurance is required if symptoms are mild. When the lesions are painful, steroids may be applied. An antiplaque mouthwash will help keep the teeth clean if brushing is painful.

What is the outlook?
Lesions in the mouth can persist for many years, much longer than any lesions that affect the skin. There is a 1 percent chance that lichen planus may show malignant change, so it is wise for a dentist to keep the disease under review.

PERICORONITIS
Inflammation of the gum that partly covers an erupting or impacted tooth, often a wisdom tooth.

Pericoronitis is a localized inflammatory condition of the gum. It usually affects young adults as the wisdom teeth in the lower jaw are erupting. If the wisdom teeth have insufficient room to erupt or are impacted into either the bone of the jaw or the tooth in front, the problem may persist for many years.

What is the cause?
A breach in the gum as the wisdom tooth erupts or attempts to erupt causes the problem. The resultant gum flap may be particularly difficult to clean, and the inflammation will become more pronounced. An opposing tooth may also irritate the area on biting and eating.

What are the symptoms?
Soreness or pain from the affected flap of gum. In severe cases, an abscess may form and there can be difficulty in opening the mouth.

How is it diagnosed?
The signs and symptoms make diagnosis straightforward. An X ray is required to determine the position of both the problematic tooth and the remaining wisdom teeth.

What are the treatment options?
The acute phase is managed by cleaning below the gum flap using an irrigation solution. Any signs of infection can be managed with antibiotics. The cusps of an opposing wisdom tooth may be smoothed to prevent injury to the gum flap or the opposing tooth may be extracted. If the tooth is impacted, it may need to be removed surgically.

PERIODONTAL DISEASE
Periodontal disease, or chronic periodontitis, in its most severe form affects 12 to 15 percent of the population.

Chronic periodontitis is always preceded by gingivitis. The disease occurs when the bone and ligament fibers that support the teeth become inflamed and then dissolve. The rate of destruction varies, but if the disease is not treated, there is a risk of losing teeth during middle and old age.

What is the cause?
It is caused by dental plaque that collects on the tooth surface as a result of ineffective brushing (see Gingivitis, p. 150). In the longer term, as the pockets around the tooth develop, the plaque will occupy sites below the gum line and become more difficult to remove. Smoking aggravates chronic periodontitis, and people with diabetes appear to be susceptible.

What are the symptoms?
The symptoms of gingivitis persist. As the support of the tooth is destroyed, additional symptoms and signs are present, such as loose teeth and gaps opening between teeth

as they drift from their original positions. Abscesses may also form in the gums. These may be painful and burst, giving rise to a foul taste. Diagnosis is by examination. X rays determine how much bone has been lost.

What are the treatment options?
Improving the standard of tooth cleaning is important. The dentist will clean and remove tartar from the root surfaces. Surgery may be necessary to reshape the gums and to gain direct vision of the roots of the teeth. Extraction may be necessary for any teeth that cannot be saved.

PULPITIS
Pulpitis is inflammation of the pulp of the tooth.

The pulp of a tooth has a rich supply of blood vessels and nerves that is essentially contained within a closed chamber. When the pulp becomes inflamed, there is an increase in pressure, as well as direct stimulation of the nerve endings.

What are the causes?
The most common cause of pulpitis is dental caries (p. 147) that has spread through the dentin to the the pulp. This includes caries that may develop beneath a filling or crown. Physical damage to a tooth and chemical irritation from some filling materials may also lead to pulpitis. If large amalgam fillings are not insulated well by lining the cavity, heat transfer may also damage the pulp.

What are the symptoms?
The primary sign of pulpitis is pain. The pain may last only a short time and be in response to a cold or a sweet stimulus, symptoms that tend to suggest that the pulpitis is reversible with treatment. If untreated, irreversible pulpitis will develop with more severe symptoms such as throbbing and persistent pain made worse by a hot stimulus.

How is it diagnosed?
A clear description of the pain will help the dentist diagnose pulpitis and its nature. Hot and cold stimuli can be used on the tooth and an electrical stimulus will help determine whether the tooth has "died." Irreversible pulpitis may have spread to the tissues around the end of the root of the tooth. The tooth may then be tender or painful to a gentle tap. An X ray will show the extent of caries in the tooth and may reveal inflammatory changes in the structure of the supporting ligament and bone.

What are the treatment options?
Reversible pulpitis is treated by removing the caries or damaged filling and replacing it. The caries also needs to be removed from any tooth with irreversible pulpitis. The extent of the damage can then be assessed. Root canal therapy or extraction of the tooth are inevitable.

SALIVARY GLAND DISORDERS
Several conditions can affect the salivary glands, causing inflammation and pain.

What are the causes?
There are several possible causes of problems in the glands:
- **Obstruction** Stones may form in the glands so that when saliva starts to flow in response to food it cannot flow out of the duct. This causes swelling and pain and may lead to infection. If left untreated, an abscess may form.
- **Infection** Salivary gland infections can be caused by bacteria or viruses. The mouth is full of bacteria, and poor hygiene can lead to an increase in number, which can infect the salivary glands. The most common viral infection in children is mumps, which causes characteristic "lumps" on the side of the neck. Mumps can occur in adults, although a lump on one side of the neck in an adult is more likely to be a result of obstruction.
- **Tumor** Most salivary gland tumors are benign and painless, causing a lump in one of the glands or on the lips, palate, or cheek. All salivary gland tumors need prompt investigation. Malignant tumors (which are rare) may be aggressive and can spread along surrounding nerves, causing severe pain and loss of facial movement.
- **Other problems** Autoimmune disorders such as rheumatoid arthritis may cause enlarged salivary glands, as can HIV, diabetes, and alcohol misuse.

What are the treatment options?
Diagnosis of a salivary gland tumor relies on taking a history and performing an examination. X rays may be necessary if stones in the glands are suspected. CT scanning may be useful to confirm the presence of a tumor, and a biopsy will be taken.

An obstructed duct may be treated by dilation of the duct to allow the stone to exit. If an obstruction causes subsequent infection, antibiotics may be prescribed. Suspicious lumps in a gland are removed by surgery. Benign lumps need no additional treatment, but if malignancy is confirmed, radiation or surgery may be prescribed.

Radiation reduces the flow of saliva, which may lead to dry mouth (Xerostomia, p. 155). Malignant tumors, however, may recur, sometimes in distant sites.

SENSITIVE TEETH
Tooth pain resulting from a loss of the protective covering over the dentin.

Dentin is the sensitive tissue and, when stimulated by touch, heat, or cold, can provoke a painful response. The dentin of the crown is covered by enamel and that of the root by a thin layer of cementum. When either of these coverings wears away or if a root is exposed during surgery, the tooth may become very sensitive. Normally, the enamel of the crown meets or overlaps the uppermost part of cementum on the root, but if they don't meet or overlap, a small amount of dentin will be exposed, and this may cause pain.

Pain—varying from mild to severe—following a stimulus to the tooth surface is the main sign of sensitive teeth. This lasts only a few seconds and disappears when the stimulus is withdrawn. Mild symptoms may be managed by using desensitizing toothpaste. In more severe cases, the dentist may apply a fluoride varnish to help desensitize the tooth or paint on a resin that can be hardened using a light source. In very severe cases it might be necessary to remove the pulp and nerve of the tooth.

TEMPOROMANDIBULAR JOINT DISORDERS
A range of disorders can affect the joint between the mandible, or jaw, and the base of the skull— the temporomandibular joint (TMJ).

The TMJ is a complex joint that has a thin disk between the opposing bones of the mandible and the base of the skull. The main muscles responsible for opening and closing the jaw are closely related to parts of the mandible near the joint. Disorders that affect other joints—such as dislocation, osteoarthritis, and ankylosis—also affect the TMJ, although the most common problem by far is temporomandibular joint dysfunction syndrome.

What are the causes?
Fatigue, overstretching, and spasm of the muscles that help open and close the jaws are the most likely causes. This can be triggered by bruxism (p. 146) or loss of the back teeth, which causes the lower jaw to adopt a new position during rest and eating.

What are the symptoms?
There is often a dull but persistent pain on the affected side of the face. The pain may be particularly bad during periods of stress and anxiety and may also be associated with headaches. Opening of the jaw may be restricted. A clicking or grating noise from the joint may also be heard.

How is it diagnosed?
There is often tenderness on palpating the affected muscles. Any restriction of jaw opening or movement can be measured. Contributing factors, such as worn teeth caused by bruxism (p. 146), will help confirm the diagnosis. X rays will not reveal abnormalities but may be taken to eliminate other conditions that might affect the joints.

What are the treatment options?
Trigger factors should be identified and corrected—for example, missing teeth may be replaced. A plastic splint can be provided to wear over the teeth at night, and physical therapy and ultrasound treatment may prove helpful.

TONGUE TIE
A condition that restricts the free movement of the tip of the tongue in babies.

Tongue tie occurs when the frenum—the soft tissue connecting the tongue to the floor of the mouth—is attached too far forward on the tongue, restricting the tongue's movement. Tongue tie may cause feeding problems in babies and may affect the teeth and speech. Surgery is rarely necessary—the tie may recede—but is an option if severe feeding problems occur or if speech is delayed.

TOOTH WEAR
As more people keep their teeth into old age, tooth wear is likely to become a major problem over the next few years.

What are the causes?
The wear of teeth can be attributed to three processes: attrition, abrasion, and erosion. In many cases, two or more of these factors are present.

- **Attrition** is caused by tooth-to-tooth contact. A common cause is grinding of teeth (see Bruxism, p. 146). Missing back teeth can also lead to attrition of the front teeth that must do all the work when eating.
- **Abrasion** is caused by factors such as overenthusiastic tooth brushing, using abrasive (smokers') toothpaste, or perhaps habitual chewing of pencils or hairpins.
- **Erosion** is caused by chemicals, usually acids, such as those present in carbonated drinks and fruit juices. The stomach also contains acids, and gastrointestinal problems causing regurgitation may contribute to tooth erosion.

What are the symptoms?

Moderate to severe wear of the teeth may affect the ability to chew and eat. When the front teeth are involved, appearance is also affected. The teeth may be painful if the enamel has been worn away, exposing the dentin underneath.

The diagnosis is obvious, but identification of all of the possible contributing factors may be more difficult and the dentist relies on an accurate history from the patient.

What are the treatment options?

The emphasis must be on prevention, by making changes to the diet, for example, or by using a plastic splint to protect the teeth if bruxism is a factor. Contributing factors should be identified and corrected. Missing teeth can be replaced.

Minimal tooth wear can be monitored to see whether the management of contributing factors is having an effect. Worn tooth surfaces can be built up to some extent by adhesive fillings. More complex restoration using crowns may sometimes be indicated. When teeth are worn almost down to gum level, a denture can be provided to fit over the worn surfaces—an overdenture.

TOOTH FRACTURE
Fractures of teeth can occur at any age but are especially common in children.

Damage to the teeth may cause fractures of just the enamel, of the enamel and the dentin, or of the crown. In severe cases, the pulp of the tooth may also be involved. A fracture may also affect the root.

What is the cause?
Trauma, commonly as a result of a fall, a sports injury, or possibly a fight. The resultant fracture will depend on the magnitude and direction of the traumatic force.

What are the symptoms?
When the fracture affects the pulp or the root, the tooth will be painful. Tenderness is also likely, as is pain of the lips and face if cuts or bruising have occurred. A child who has suffered a severe blow may have lost consciousness. The child, and often the parents, will be very anxious.

How is it diagnosed?
The clinical examination needs to be supplemented by an X ray of the tooth to show the full extent of the fracture. Occasionally, a small piece of enamel might become embedded in the lip; this can also be seen on an X ray.

What are the treatment options?
Teeth with fractures that affect enamel and dentin may be built up using a tooth-colored adhesive filling. When the pulp is involved, root canal therapy is likely to be necessary. If the tooth has not fully developed, the root will not be completely formed. Part of the living pulp may be left in the root to try to encourage further growth of the tooth. When a large part of the tooth has been fractured, long-term restoration with a crown is necessary.

XEROSTOMIA
Xerostomia is a temporary or permanent dry mouth.

Dry mouth is not a disease as such but rather a single manifestation of one of a number of disorders. It is a consequence of a lack or absence of saliva in the mouth.

A state of anxiety or dehydration resulting from sweating, diarrhea, or vomiting can cause a temporary dry mouth. Dry mouth also occurs after radiation to the head and neck as part of cancer treatment when the salivary glands are in the X-ray beam. It is a feature of diabetes and may be a side effect of certain drugs, including antihistamines and antidepressants. A lump of calculus in the main duct of one of the salivary glands may also reduce saliva flow into the mouth.

Dry mouth varies in severity. When the saliva is virtually absent, the lining of the mouth becomes red and inflamed. The patient may also complain of a burning mouth. The cause of the dry mouth must be identified and treated. Artificial saliva substitutes are available, but some patients find that frequently sipping water is effective. A persistent dry mouth will increase the risk of tooth decay, so regular dental checkups are recommended.

Index

Acknowledgments

Carroll & Brown Limited would also like to thank:

Picture researcher
Sandra Schneider

Production manager
Karol Davies

Production controller
Nigel Reed

Computer management
Paul Stradling

Indexer
Jill Dormon

3D anatomy
Mirashade/Matt Gould

Illustrators
Andy Baker, Rajeev Doshi/Regraphica, Jacey, Kevin Jones Associates, Mikki Rain, John Woodcock

Layout and illustration assistance
Joanna Cameron

Photographers
Jules Selmes, David Yems

Photographic sources
SPL = Science Photo Library

1 Omikron/SPL
6 *(right)* Getty Images
7 Zephyr/SPL
8 *(top left)* Bill Longcore/SPL
9 *(top left)* Bob Krist/Corbis
10 *(top)* BSIP, Kretz Technik/SPL
(bottom right) Jules Selmes
11 *(top)* Alex Bartel/SPL
(bottom) Getty Images
12 *(top)* Bill Longcore/SPL
(bottom) Lauren Shear/SPL
13 *(top)* A. Crump,TDR,WHO/SPL
(bottom) Volker Steger,
Peter Arnold Inc/SPL
14 *(left)* Getty Images
(right) Custom Medical Stock Photo/SPL
25 Omikron/SPL
27 Custom Medical Stock Photo/SPL
28 Prof. P. Motta/G. Franchitto/ University "La Sapienza" Rome/SPL
36 *(center)* Getty Images
(bottom) Michael S. Yamashita/ Corbis
37 Getty Images
38 *(left)* L. Clarke/Corbis
40 *(left, top right)* Getty Images

(2nd from top) Jose Luis Pelaez Inc./Corbis
(3rd from top) Jim Craigmyle/ Corbis
(5th from top) Getty Images
41, 43, 45 Getty Images
46 Jose Luis Pelaez Inc./Corbis
48 Getty Images
50 *(top)* John Birdsall Photography
(2nd from top) Getty Images
52 Jim Craigmyle/Corbis
55, 56 Getty Images
63 *(3rd from top right)* Getty Images
64 *(left)* Robert Judges/Rex Features
(center) Getty Images
(right) Jon Feingersh/Corbis
65 *(left)* L. Clarke/Corbis
69 *(center right)* Getty Images
(bottom) Michael Keller/Corbis
70, 71 *(top)* Getty Images
71 *(center)* George Shelley/Corbis
(bottom) Karl Weatherley/Corbis
72, 73 Getty Images
78 *(top right)* Michael Busselle/Corbis
(3rd from top) Getty Images
80 *(center right)* Getty Images
(bottom right) Michael Busselle/ Corbis
81 TH Foto-Werbung/SPL
85 Getty Images
90 *(left)* George Bernard/SPL
(center) Alex Bartel/SPL
(right) CC Studio/SPL
91 Mediscan
94 Getty Images
96 Adam Hart-Davies/SPL
97 *(left)* CC Studio/SPL
(top right) Don Wong/SPL
(bottom right) BSIP Kokel/SPL
98 Andrew McClenaghan/SPL
99 *(top left)* Dr. P. Marazzi/SPL
(bottom) Argentum/SPL
102 BSIP, Chassenet/SPL
103 Wellcome Trust Medical Photographic Library
104 *(top left)* MIG/medipics
(bottom left, right) Diane Hodds/ medipics
105 Mediscan
106 Kevin Harrison/medipics
108 *(top, center)* Dr. P. Marazzi/SPL
(bottom) Hank Morgan/SPL
109 *(top)* BSIP, Laurent/SPL
(center, center right, bottom) Dr. P. Marazzi/SPL
(inset) Klaus Guldbrandsen/SPL
110 St. Bartholomew's Hospital, London/SPL

111 *(top left, center)* Dr. P. Marazzi/SPL
(bottom) Lauren Shear/SPL
116 Tom Stewart/Corbis
118 *(left)* Ken Eward/SPL
(right) George Bernard/SPL
121 Volker Steger/SPL
123 *(top)* SPL
(bottom) Dr. Peter Gordon
124 *(top)* Alex Bartel/SPL
(bottom) Oscar Burriel/SPL
127 *(left)* Zephyr/SPL
128 *(top)* Maximilian Stock Ltd/SPL
129 *(left)* Carolyn A. McKeone/SPL
(right) Alex Bartel/SPL
130 Dr. Peter Gordon
131 *(top)* Dr. P. Marazzi/SPL
(bottom) Eamonn McNulty/SPL
132 Tony McConnell/SPL

Back cover *(right)* St. Bartholomew's Hospital, London/SPL

Items for photography on pages 50–51 loaned by RNIB, London

Contact details
American Academy of Periodontology
www.perio.org

American Dental Association
www.ada.org

American Diabetes Association
www.diabetes.org

American Association of Orthodontists
www.braces.org

National Association for Parents of Children with Visual Impairments (NAPVI)
www.spedex.com

National Federation of the Blind
800 Johnson Street
Baltimore, MD 21230
1-410-659-9314
www.nfb.org

National Library Service for the Blind and Physically Handicapped (NLS)
www.loc.gov/nls